"Jacob has walked with me th... my life. As a coach, he compass... ... persevere while providing support when those days arose that felt insurmountable. I wouldn't be where I am today without Jacob's guidance. I have told my family and friends—if you want to reevaluate where you are, take a step in the right direction, or just aren't sure what the future may bring, schedule time with Jacob and make him part of your success plan."

—Tyler Dunphy, Senior Director,
TPx Communications, Maine

"Without Jacob, the six-figure success we experienced in our first year of business would not have been possible. His methods are practical, his advice is actionable, and his approach is personable. I cannot recommend him highly enough."

—Tanner Campbell,
Owner of The Portland Pod, Maine

"Jacob's coaching came at crucial cross-roads in my life, both professionally and personally. His patient and thoughtful process along with his ability to help me get to the root of 'me' has been invaluable to my life. Within a very short time, my increased production paid for his services ten-fold. Both my wife and I are very thankful for Jacob's help in focusing me on what's really important. Thanks Jacob, for making me more profitable in every sense of the word."

—Jon Taylor, National Sales and Training Director,
CU Certified Automotive, Maine

At a crucial time in my business, Jacob led me on a path to really search within to focus on what matters most in my life. His approach helped save time, money, and most importantly, helped me be a better husband, father, and person.

—Dr. Mitchell Vance,
Owner of Body Back Chiropractic and Physiotherapy, Maine

"Jacob, I see now how I had never stopped to observe how I was making decisions for my business. With your guidance I came to see I'd been investing in too many places to try and produce growth. In learning from our coaching around Compass Form, I came to see that there were better uses of my time and energy that didn't cost me any money and built word-of-mouth referrals. Since then, I have more clients than I can handle myself and have brought on board a salaried employee. Thanks for providing this insight and tool for me to use and simplify life."

—Victor Rios,
Owner of Expose Design, Maine

"Working with Jacob has been incredibly valuable to my business, family life, and mental and physical health. I've learned more about who I am, what I value, and how to react to stressful situations in a productive manner and embrace the next obstacle. Most importantly, Jacob has helped me feel OK about where I am, confident on where I'm going, and comfortable with the fact that there will be bumps along the road. If you're running a business built on real human relationships and struggling to find a balance between work and family, I highly recommend working with Jacob and Compass Form. You owe it to yourself, your family, and your clients. You'll be glad you did."

—Adam Rothbart, CRPC,
Integrated Financial Planners, Maine

BEFORE 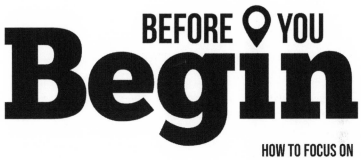 YOU
Begin

HOW TO FOCUS ON
WHAT MATTERS AND
GET THE LIFE YOU WANT

JACOB COLDWELL

To my wife, Kristin, and our children, McKenzie, Ezra, and Ezekiel for walking this road with me.

And to Mom and Dad for introducing to me what a commitment is, 50 years and counting.

And to my brother Mac.

"Life ultimately means taking the responsibility to find the right answer to its problems and to fulfill the tasks which it constantly sets for each individual."

—*Man's Search for Meaning*
by Viktor E. Frankl

JACOB'S GIFT TO YOU: COMPASS FORM EMAIL COURSE!

Before you begin your journey reading *Before You Begin*, go to https://themountainpassway.com/emailcourse to access the free email course Jacob developed to give you further guidance using the tools he presents in this book. This course provides additional resources, exercises, and tools to focus on what matters and get the life you want.

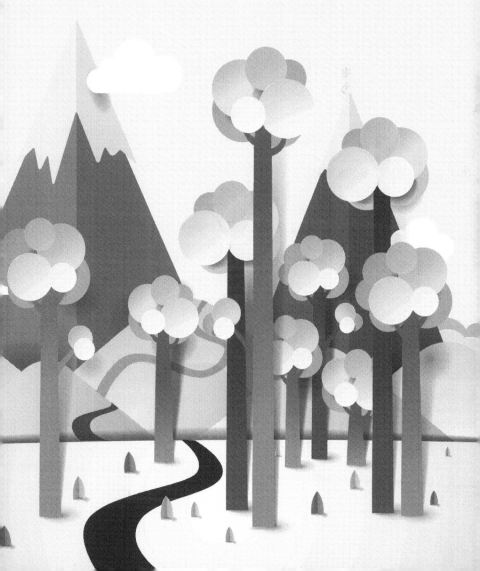

CONTENTS

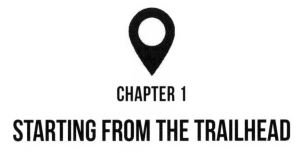

CHAPTER 1

STARTING FROM THE TRAILHEAD

"If the journey is the destination, then we must learn how to become better travelers. To become better travelers, we must first learn to orient ourselves. Where are you now? Do you want to be here? If not, why do you want to move on?"

— *The Bullet Journal Method*
by Ryder Carroll

If you were going to take a road trip, where would you go? How would you go? Would you get in the car and take off? Would you create lists and plan for weeks, making sure to notify everyone you know that you won't be around for a while? Would you take the safest route? The fastest route? The most picturesque route even if it was a bit isolated? Would you get stuck trying to decide on where you want to end up?

A trip to the store is familiar enough to allow us to get into the car and drive. But a trip across the country would be a much greater endeavor. It requires a bit more planning and uncertainty, as there are many miles between here and the destination. There are mandatory off-ramps to refuel and take breaks. It is never as simple as getting in the car and driving. There are a few things that need to happen Before You Begin any journey.

As with a cross-country road trip, our own intention is the only reliable gauge that can keep us on course to a life that brings us significance. But why in our own life do we live distracted from our intention? Why are we looking for others to approve our choices and agree with our plans? Why are we living lives that don't mean that much to us?

When you think about how you make decisions for your family, career, interests, relationships, health, and such, you can take a lot from the road trip comparison. From wherever you are at this point, there are a number of steps that fill the gap between starting and reaching where you want to go. The problem is that you can lose your way between here and there. There are twists and turns that you don't see coming, and those unexpected forks can create bumps that throw you off course. The ultimate goal of this book is to help you keep your eyes on the road and to show you how anything less than being aware and intentional creates obstacles that prevent you from staying the course.

In order to have a life that will have meaning, you will have to find purpose in what you do. While few circumstances are controllable, you always have the capacity to take what life gives and live it on your own terms. How you want to show up and step forward in life is always in your control. Giving yourself the capacity to focus on what matters amidst the chaos that shows up in life is an invaluable tool. *Before You Begin* locates this tool for you and teaches you how to use it.

Before You Begin provides a flexible framework, so you can quickly assess and settle on the task at hand, so then you can drive. So you can move through the endless distractions and enjoy your journey. It's about forgetting where you just came from because you have already been there and done that. It's about having enough confidence to trust that the destination you've chosen is worth committing to, and it's about knowing that uncertainty before arrival is part of the plan.

Settling on a few things Before You Begin heading down the road will not only get you to where you want to go, but will give you an optimal experience to navigate the changes that are certain to show up. Without *Before You Begin*, life's inevitable problems, frustrations, and discomforts can totally rattle you. So much so that you might get twisted and bent and start reacting without thinking. You lose your way. You end up giving up on your ideal just to make it through the day. You find yourself stuck, stagnant, hustling in circles, and exhausted, but getting nowhere. This exhaustion, stagnancy, and lostness can play out in a myriad of ways. Here are some "stuck" situations that my clients have found themselves in that could ring true for you too:

- Your job sucks and waking up every day is miserable. You've had three jobs in the past three years, and they all looked promising until you start working at each one. You don't even like what you do, but it pays the bills. You live for the end of the day. And for the weekend. Starting over seems like way too much work for no guarantee of happiness.

- You have a bucket list, but nothing is getting checked off. Traveling to Europe, jumping out of an airplane, starting your own consulting company, or buying your first guitar and learning to play your favorite song—you never seem to be able to find the time to fit these life goals in.

- You want to grow your business. You've tried a multitude of courses, seminars, read books, and participated in pricey mastermind groups. You've put a lot of ideas into action, but it just isn't working.

- You recently got divorced and want to start dating again. You've read some self-help books on the subject and taken lots of advice from friends, family, and colleagues. You've even gone on some dates. But it hasn't been going well.

- Your doctor has warned you about your weight and your health, and though you're trying—you've listened to health podcasts, read books about bettering your health, tried changing your diet and regularly exercising—nothing sticks.

- You know you commit to way too much. The schedule you have keeps you rushing from one promise to another. You are constantly letting people down by showing up late and missing out on the relationships that you love. You are spread so thin that no one really knows you anymore. You don't know yourself anymore. But you can't say no, especially to something good.

Similar to the people in these examples, if you've been trying to change an aspect of your life for the better—but no matter how much you try, you find yourself stuck—then this book is for you. *Before You Begin* provides you a simple and flexible framework from which to operate so that you can move from a place of stagnancy to take a step forward to where you want to go. This book helps you establish the foundation to operate from before you take any actions. You see, before you engage with any programs, courses, books, coaches, seminars, or mastermind groups, for any of those to be effective, you need to have an idea of where you are heading Before You Begin.

Before You Begin guides you to change the way you are currently engaging the world so that you can experience different results. Results that align with what you intend as opposed to reacting to whatever happens in each moment. In order to begin creating a new habit, *Before You Begin*'s framework allows you a simple way to recognize and create new paths to think about situations where you do not yet have an answer. Compass Form is the name of this book's framework.

YOUR COMPASS, NOT YOUR MAP

Compass Form is a framework for you to organize the chaos so that you can take an action step. Compass Form is not about building a plan. It is a process to keep you moving in a sensible direction. It gives you the ability to be wise and flexible because your attention goes to what you can control, even though life shifts quickly. It also allows you to get somewhere because it allows you to see life for what it is (as opposed to how you might imagine, hope, or fear it to be) and make an adjustment to control what you can. It allows you to quickly ground yourself in the moment you feel lost, so you can return focus on where to place your next step and then act.

As the name implies, Compass Form supports you in a way similar to a compass. It will not tell you exactly where to go or what you should do—as a map or set of directions would. But, like a compass, it simply clarifies where you are and where you want to go overall, so that you can decide the next step to take that orients you in your decided direction.

Unlike a set of directions or a map, life isn't clear. Life's journey moves and shifts. Plans can break down and become chaotic in a moment. A compass allows you to be present to your present circumstances and to any unforeseen problems long enough to understand them and navigate them. The compass points you in the direction of your overall aim. It helps you to wisely move, even without seeing every future step in the entire journey. The compass points you in the direction you know you want to head. It helps you to move around obstacles that don't appear on a map. This framework assists you to create a clear direction when you lose touch with your life.

Compass Form is about isolating decisions, so you address them specifically and clear some of the chaos that comes with trying to make many decisions at once or trying to make the "perfect" decision. It isn't about predicting the future. Life is ambiguous and chaotic. The skill that is being built is learning how to quickly make sense of the chaos and being content with the best decision possible given the reality of your circumstances. Compass Form allows you to navigate uncertainty, settle on a decision, and at the same time regularly adjust your course. That's what you'll learn to do in this book.

Once you establish and become adept at engaging Compass Form in your life, that's when you will finally make progress in your journey from where you are to where you want to go.

ME AND COMPASS FORM

Who am I? Why should you listen to me? As you'll soon read in this book, I am someone who found myself stuck and frustrated—in a 12-year rut. While my personal life was pretty good, it was my career that remained stagnant. I was running my own business, but it didn't carry the satisfaction and meaningfulness that I'd hoped it would—and I couldn't get out or change that. I tried and tried for over 12 years, but nothing seemed to be working. Though it was debilitating at the time, the framework for emerging from stagnancy—Compass Form—developed from that period and pointing myself in the direction of success and satisfaction came about.

While it seemed frustrating and impossible, through my own pursuit of growing myself in order to live a life of meaning, I came upon several insights that culminated in Compass Form. Though I don't have a map for success, I found a compass that I used (and continue to use) to orient myself, so I can continue in the direction of success and satisfaction. Over seven years ago, I got out of this stuckness and started my dream job: I became a personal coach. Since then, I've guided others out of their stagnancy, so they too can progress to their particular direction of success. Compass Form is the foundational framework that I teach my clients to use to progress to success and satisfaction. Let me share with you the story of one of my clients, Victor.

In early 2019, I was introduced to Victor Rios, owner of Expose Design in Maine. We started talking about the struggles he had been facing with growing his business and getting it to another level. He was a solopreneur who was about five years into being a full-time logo designer. After working through the principles of Compass Form, Victor shared this with me:

"Jacob, I see now how I had never stopped to observe how I was making decisions for my business. With your guidance I came to see I'd been investing in too many places to try and produce growth. I'd thought spending money on marketing, rather than utilizing my current client base, would fix the problem of leveling off. In learning from our coaching around Compass Form, I came to see that there were better uses of my

time and energy that didn't cost me any money and built word-of-mouth referrals. Since then, I have more clients than I can handle myself and have brought on board a salaried employee, plus commission, as an incentive for any new customers the employee can produce. If someone had spoken to me before my coaching with you, I would have argued, "Why pay someone to do what I can do?" But I realize now that I'm not paying someone to do what I can do. I'm investing in someone to help grow my business, and as a bonus, it has saved me time, which is more valuable to me than any dollar amount. Why? Because now I have more time to focus on business development, family life, and my health and wellness. Thanks for providing this insight and tool for me to use and simplify life."

OVERVIEW OF *BEFORE YOU BEGIN*

The journey of *Before You Begin* starts with my story and how I remained stuck for so long, yearning for a different career and trying everything with nothing ever quite working. I start with my story because what I've gone through is similar to so many others wanting to make progress but not finding success. The aim of giving my story is for readers to recognize their own struggles, patterns of frustration, and reactionary ways of dealing—but you'll find more than that. I also outline how I stumbled upon and put into effect what I now call Compass Form to finally get my feet out of the mire and make progress, one step at a time, to a career that I find meaningful. As I mentioned, I'm now a life coach, a dream job that is chocked full of challenge and meaning—what I'd been yearning for, but pre-Compass Form wasn't able to effect.

After that, we launch into Compass Form. You'll get a close look at what this approach to life is and what it is not. Through comparisons, examples, reflection questions, and exercises—that you'll find in every chapter starting in chapter 2—you'll get to reflect on your own patterns of thinking and acting that have likely kept you stagnant and far from progressing closer to your goals, whether those goals be in terms of your health, career, marriage, etc. You'll also get plenty of content to increase your understanding of Compass Form.

After that we delve into how to enact Compass Form in your life. How to engage it as your approach to living. Because Compass Form manifests in three steps—observe, focus, and act—we spend time parsing these concepts. Again, you'll get plenty of example scenarios, questions, and practical activities so that you are equipped to engage Compass Form in your life in order to finally get out of stagnation and frustration and start making real progress toward where you want to be. At any point in this book, if you have a question, idea, or you decide you want to explore getting one-on-one guidance in engaging Compass Form in your own life, please contact me— jacob@themountainpassway.com and https://themountainpassway. com. I am available for you.

ORGANIZE THE CHAOS TO FINALLY PROGRESS!

The truth is, you can't and don't know everything about what lies ahead. You can't control all the steps you will need to take. You can only decide if you want to take the steps that will get you to where you want to go.

What you'll find in *Before You Begin* is that you quickly move from chaos and confusion to making a sensible decision that will change something in your life. It allows you to find what is currently important, even in the midst of many demands coming at you, so you can get closer to what matters; even when you're not certain on exactly what that is yet. It guides you to break down any complexity into a simple and tangible action. When you combine consistent steps and your intention stays true, then the end results in what you wanted to see happen.

In the next chapter I'll show you what Compass Form can look like from my own story. The point is to help you see another way to engage your life, not to look at my life as a model of success for you to emulate. Another reason for sharing my story is to show you what living proof looks like when a person enacts Compass Form in hopes that you'll get the inspiration and motivation to engage it.

It's time to get out your compass! Turn the page to get started in orientating yourself in your unique direction of success.

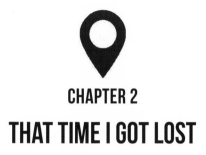

CHAPTER 2
THAT TIME I GOT LOST

"People think they think, but it's not true. It's mostly self-criticism that passes for thinking. True thinking is rare—just like true listening. Thinking is listening to yourself. It's difficult. To think, you have to be at least two people at the same time. Then you have to let those people disagree. Thinking is an internal dialogue between two or more different views of the world."

— *12 Rules for Life: An Antidote to Chaos*
by Jordan B. Peterson

To comprehend the Compass Form framework, see how it works, and get pumped to engage it in your own life, we start by looking at what Compass Form is and what it is not. You'll read how I lived and engaged with life before Compass Form and then after. While my story may not be exactly like yours on the surface, underneath people are pretty similar, so I expect my story is one you'll be able to identify with in its overarching struggles and ultimately its victories. As you read, I encourage you to note how I was stuck and where you might currently be. Consider if and how the cage of thinking and behavioral patterns that describe my stagnancy pertain to you too. And when I share how I managed to emerge and bridge the gap from where I was—stuck and/or moving in random circles—to where I wanted to be—moving forward towards a career of meaningful work—that's what came to be Compass Form. Notice how my mindset started changing once I landed upon key insights that led to Compass Form.

ME AND MY "STUCKNESS"

Near the end of my twenties, I had been living a string of days that had turned into years of trying to find what I wanted to do with my life. At the time I had been building a painting business, and it wasn't working out the way I had hoped.

I had ideas that I would start a painting service and grow it into a business. Problem was I had never owned a business and was naive about what owning a business meant. After a few years, I figured out a few things and faced one major problem that impacted how much I could grow the business: I didn't want employees. After hiring a few people, I recognized I was spending too much time trying to get people to paint my way. I was rechecking their work, and all this added more to my plate. I didn't have the capacity to paint and train at the same time. I found that when working on my own, I could make as much income and avoid the complications of having other people to be responsible for. For me, to keep life simple was of more importance than building a bigger business.

For the next decade, I had to work every day to make enough to pay the bills for our family of five. My amazing wife took on the majority of managing the family. Although she saved us an enormous amount of money, we still needed income to come in, and that was on me.

We were always trying to keep our heads above water financially. We learned to sacrifice to keep the lifestyle that fit our family, with my wife managing the home and me bringing in the income. We sold things we didn't need. We limited how often we would go out to eat. At one point we attempted to live with one car although that experiment didn't last long.

The decision to live as a family of five off one income was our choice, but it came with a cost and sacrifice we never knew to consider when we started out. We weren't able to take time off or have vacations. It wasn't until about ten years of painting that we finally were able to take our first real family trip. Five days driving down to Hershey, Pennsylvania, and then on to Williamsburg, Virginia.

I was working hard, but the results of that work only kept us floating above water financially. It was awful and stressful. Our livelihood was based on steady work, and there was no room for a gap. And the work became mundane. Day after day, I'd creep out of bed, throw on some crappy clothes and prepare to head out to the next job. Basically, I came to hate my job, and I felt shackled to it.

I knew that if I didn't make a certain amount each week, then we would not have enough. We learned to live week to week with the uncertainty of what might happen the following week. These **fears** filled my mind during the day. **The fear would spin out of control** on the good days, and the bad days they would rip out my insides and take what motivation I had left.

I would keep needling the same thoughts over and over. *Will the work keep coming in? What if I get sick? How can I get out of this rut? How long can I physically keep this up?*

Work, home, sleep. Repeat. I put myself in this position and made the choices years earlier, but the dream I had started with turned into a recurring nightmare. A boring and detached life with no real hope of change.

It was exhausting to carry the burden of providing for my family and fearing what would happen if I failed. It was worse to tackle it alone. Days began to run together. By the end of my work as a painter, I used the same process to paint over 2,500 rooms. The rest of the math was too depressing.

The problem was that I was **reacting** to life. I was waiting for life to happen and then trying to manage the results with whatever wisdom and experience I remembered in the moment. Life happened to me, and I felt like I could never make changes or live a life that I would enjoy. I had to take care of my family, and this was the only way to make it happen.

I didn't come to resolve my miserable life without a fight. I was constantly reading and trying new ideas. On average I was reading 40 books a year. I took courses and trainings to learn new skills and find another opportunity to get out of painting. I ended up with college-level certificates in project management and missional leadership. Later on, I would get certified as a life coach and StoryBrand Certified Guide.

I didn't sit around only chewing on my thoughts and licking my wounds, I was searching for an answer to what I should be and do with my life. But I had no real idea.

I naturally spend a lot of time thinking. I joke with people and classify myself as a "high-functioning severely introverted" person. I spent hours noodling through whatever came to mind each day as I dipped another brush-load of paint to cover the crappy wall that I was going to "transform"!

I spent over 12 years in the job, and I didn't enjoy the work. By the time I was able to walk away, I had long since used the fumes of what fuel of motivation there was and was merely rolling to a stop.

A CRUCIAL REALIZATION: THE ILLUSION OF CONTROL

At around the five-year mark, I learned something so valuable.

You can't control life.

I typically would hit a slow patch around the winter season, as people aren't looking to get much work done on their homes around the holidays. However, one particular such winter stretch was a bit longer than what I had experienced before, and we had run out of money. Bills were coming in, and there wasn't anything left to pay them with.

Being self-employed has some drawbacks. Banks look at you as riskier than traditionally employed people. So we ended up having to cash out what was left of our 401k to make it to the next week.

I had nothing left to control. I was working my butt off trying to make life work out—trying to control life—and I was getting nowhere close to it. It was exhausting to try to keep this life running. There was no way I could keep this up for however many years I had left to live—60, 40, 20? Who knew? But it really didn't matter.

In my mind, this wasn't a life worth living.

So there was a choice to make. Either I keep the same approach and expectations for life and more than likely experience the same results, or I give up this approach for another way. But I didn't know another way to go about engaging in life. Even still, it was clear that this way wasn't working, and I could not continue in the same manner.

I chose to give up this approach that wasn't working.

Before, my assumption had been that if I could determine the "best" answers" and the "perfect" plan, I would avoid making big mistakes—I would be in control. But when I looked back at my life, what I didn't see was a bunch of great choices and amazing outcomes. I had a few good outcomes and avoided some bad ones, but even still, I had many more less-than-ideal outcomes than major victories. I'd never recognized this before. For me, it had always been easier to remember the successes and run past what didn't work out.

That showed me two things:
1. **I wasn't as good of a decision-maker as I imagined.**
2. **The decisions didn't have as much value as I'd given them.**

It was a major eyeopener to begin to see that there were other ways to live and to think about how I approached the world. There were always a lot of choices to make, but I thought they had to go through my way of processing so that I could make them work out, i.e., so I could (seemingly) control and dictate the outcomes.

Later on in life I found this Viktor Frankl quote that pretty well summarizes the realization of where I was at: "When we are no longer able to change a situation—just think of an incurable disease such as inoperable cancer—we are challenged to change ourselves."

The only way I found to change myself was to give up my way of making choices and decisions.

Before, my premise had been that I was in control of all decisions and making them work out the way I thought they needed to go. Assuming this premise to be true had been my biggest problem. I would have to let go of this premise—the assumption that I could control things and that I could make the "perfect" decision—a truth that I'd long held. I'd have to change my whole approach to life and begin with something new.

I didn't know what other options there were to approach life. For almost 30 years I had made decisions using one approach, so to leave that approach was of monumental proportions. It was both frightening and freeing at the same time.

I had a responsibility, but—based on my big realization—I didn't need to try so hard to be (or feel like I was) in control.

MORE ON OUR LACK OF TOTAL CONTROL

When I looked at just percentages, maybe 25% of things I worked on ended up turning out how I thought they should. Those are not good odds, but they do indicate that though I'd thought I could control outcomes through my decisions, 75% of the time—most of the time—I couldn't. I was under the illusion I was in control. Upon clearly seeing this, I started working on finding a new way.

I began to look outside my own head for other ways to approach decisions that needed to be made. What I found was that the world around me had always played more of a role than I was aware of. I wasn't in control of outcomes. I didn't control the minds of anyone or anything. I didn't control the weather. I didn't control the economy.

I didn't control politics. I didn't control the personalities, moods, and circumstances of my family, friends, clients, and others in my community. I didn't control traffic. I didn't control the amount of time in a day, the rising and setting of the sun, the rotation of the planets around the sun and the moon around the earth. Sure, I could decide when to wake up and when to sleep, but even then my mind or body could refuse to fall asleep.

And here is the freedom—I didn't need to approach the way I lived as if I controlled every single thing in order to exist—and exist well—in the world. I learned that I existed in a much larger world than what I was aware of. It's like pulling the curtain open and seeing outside a room you'd been living in for decades. I had locked myself inside an imaginary house, and I thought my only job was to protect it.

Trying to maintain control was like carrying a home, trying to hold it up, but getting crushed and exhausted over and over again from the effort. But the reality always was that it never was trying to destroy me. I was pushing up against an imaginary wall that didn't need me to support it. Life existed without me for many years before I was born. It continued on, whether I was pushing on it or not.

Because of this, my own world was no longer dependent on me. I was free to look at new ways to engage life. But that was also scary. I'd never operated in this manner.

It is unfamiliar territory to allow life to happen without trying to leverage it to meet your own design. Even though, if you really think about it, this is what is happening anyway, meaning thinking that you are controlling and designing everything is a burdensome illusion.

SCENIC OVERLOOK

- No matter how much we resist, ignore, or act otherwise, we can't control life.
- When we operate from the premise that somehow we can control life, we unnecessarily place a huge burden on ourselves.
- There is freedom in realizing we can't control life.

PERSONAL DECLINATION

- What is an area of life where you would like to see a change?
- What specifically do you know to be true in this situation?
- What is causing or contributing to you wanting the change?
- What has been keeping you from the ideal outcome that you want to change to?
- After running through these questions, how is your view of the situation changing?

OUT-AND-BACK EXERCISE

Take one small change you'd like to make in your life that hasn't worked out yet and try to approach it in a new way.

For example: when I attend a conference or training, my comfortable way to show up is to sit back and avoid conversation. I changed my mindset and introduced myself to people when it seemed to fit. In doing so, I was able to build relationships that I would not have been able to, simply because I expressed what I was hoping others would do for me. What I learned is that I experienced something different as a result of initiating, and it was also authentic because I was selective. But the main point was that because I initiated a change, I experienced different results.

Here are some ideas on areas where you could experiment with making a small change: getting to the gym, cleaning a cluttered room, eating out less or more, etc.

After a few attempts, reflect on what you experienced and write down some takeaways.

- Did you see different results? How did you feel before?
- After?
- What might you do differently next time? Is there a big enough return to continue with your change?

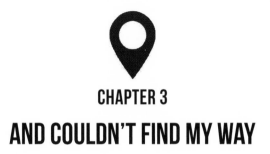

CHAPTER 3
AND COULDN'T FIND MY WAY

"Learn to follow a compass and you won't be wandering aimlessly around in circles. Walk in a straight line, and you may eventually find a familiar landmark, a road to rescue, or a place to ask for help."

— *Be Expert with Map and Compass*
by Bjorn Kjellstrom and Carina Kjellstrom Elgin

This chapter continues to relate my journey to changing my approach to life. Even though the previous chapter left off with my coming upon some major insights, it didn't translate to a quick "happily ever after." But this is normal. Of course we want to experience immediate positive results, but often they don't come as soon as we hope. Good change doesn't necessarily correlate to an enjoyable, easy experience. Sometimes when a rock is kicked over, what is underneath isn't pretty.

In this chapter, you'll see that even when growth takes place, it doesn't mean the struggle is over. Even still, it doesn't mean we're wrong or should turn around. We should aim to notice the importance of staying the course and not basing our choices on immediate results. We will succeed eventually, so it's important that we don't celebrate, or expect to celebrate, too soon. The goal isn't getting to an easy life; it's to be confident in creating the life we believe should exist for ourselves, no matter the cost. Let's look at how this played out for me.

STUCK IN PURGATORY

I had already begun the process to try and get away from painting as a career. One option I tried was to pursue becoming a pastor. This career change—as was true of any change I endeavored to make—I had to seek outside (or, in addition to) my full-time painting work. It was a risk for me to try and leverage what little money was available to hopefully prompt a different course.

To become a pastor, I enrolled into a correspondence certificate program. How it worked is that after working a full day, I would come home and read and write. Once a month I would fly out to Seattle for the weekend to meet with fellow students to process and learn more.

Also I started looking for opportunities to volunteer or become a paid staff at local churches. But it never went very far. When you throw being a painter and having a master's certificate on a resume as your life experience for becoming a pastor, there aren't too many people with the imagination to think that is a good idea. On top of that I didn't have the chops of a four-year degree or seminary or a long history of leadership positions in the church.

Something I learned in pursuing becoming a pastor was that you had to do what you wanted to become. It was the chicken and egg reality. You can't get a job without experience, and you can't get experience without a job. It didn't make sense to hand over a position like being a pastor to someone who had no proof of concept.

As I began to implement becoming more pastoral, I had to guess at what to work on personally to begin creating some proof of experience. For the first time I had to question how I was brought up with how I wanted to show up and approach everyday life. I looked at the way I was living and began contrasting it with this new information to make sure things were lining up. After a few attempts at trying to find work as a pastor over the next year, I gave up on that dream.

Although this didn't end in the success I had hoped for, which was a new life without painting, it created a change internally that gave me more perspective and insight. It was during this time I started to learn the first part of the Compass Form framework: **observe**. At the time, what looked dismal and a failure actually had a lot more to it. I was looking for a certain result going into this career change, and I assessed failure to it because I didn't run across that finish line.

What I failed to see at the time was that in one dream dying a new one was birthed. At that time I didn't consider other options regarding what was taking place. I was stuck on becoming a pastor or not, and if I did not, I'd failed. However, in time, something rose from the ashes of that experience. It was a refined insight that showed me more about myself and what purpose I could have in this world.

"Observe" is about taking inventory on what is true. Not what we want to be true.

In my aim to become a pastor, I had in mind an imaginary picture of what that life should be. It wasn't real, just a figment of my

imagination, but I gave a lot of credence to it. It wasn't effective to make decisions in real life by using a made-up dream as the foundation. This dream notion of what I imagined a pastor's life to be was what I thought was best for me, but how on earth was that even valid? Especially as it was an idealized notion, laden with "shoulds" and "supposed tos."

What I eventually came to realize is that I didn't enjoy preaching and sharing messages to people from the center of a stage. That wasn't comfortable for me. I wasn't at my best in that setup. I was an introvert trying to force my way into a bad opportunity. Something that was outside of myself that I was trying to force my way through.

And I learned that even though the summation of becoming a pastor didn't work out, it also wasn't a waste. In my efforts to change, I found out something about how I saw the world. I saw that I enjoyed listening to people. I recognized I liked seeing people change and grow in maturity. I found that life was a bit more meaningful for me when I could do some of these things I was enjoying.

When I was able to reconcile the benefit from the failure, it was easier to let go of the idea of being a pastor as I'd originally envisioned it. In the meantime, **the truth about not being in control was changing my perspective beyond just my career path. It was changing how I perceived everything.**

It's odd because what was visible on the outside wasn't changing much. I was still painting. In the off hours of reading and learning, I was finding how to be a better listener to others. However, subconsciously my realization that control is an illusion was affecting a lot more of me. It changed my relationship with my wife, with my kids, and with people that I would share life with. I could hear more than just the words they spoke, and it opened the way to me being able to help them out.

As this new idea of living started to build and become more familiar, I continued consuming information at a high level. I read a lot. I liked learning about how to get unstuck in my own life. In the past ten years, I have read over 500 books and counting. You could say I am a slow learner, but I prefer the term "thorough learner." Quite honestly, I learned a lot on my own. I listened to friends I have never met but who were willing to share their wisdom and experience through their writing. The more I read, the more I could try to change.

As I continued to look into making changes, I stumbled on one of the most impactful books I had ever read. It was a book on listening. Now if you asked me before I read this book, I would have answered that listening is something I thought I was proficient at. Right here is a lesson that would repeat itself. Just because I have done something many times doesn't mean I know what I am doing. I thought I had a good handle on listening, but as I was reading the book, another level opened up that I'd never considered. It added new options to choose from and showed me that the wisdom I had was immature as there were deeper levels of listening. Letting go of the past allowed me to consider more options that, otherwise, I would have dismissed, thinking I was proficient.

This has happened a few times for me. For example, a few years back, I started working with a nutritionist. I was gaining weight and didn't want it to continue. I had been running for a few years, but it wasn't enough to keep me from adding on pounds.

When I met with the nutritionist, I quickly learned that there was more to eating than just putting food in my mouth. I had been eating on my own for almost 40 years, and in ten minutes of working with the nutritionist, I knew I didn't know how to eat. I'd never given it thought before. I'd assumed because I ate often that I was good at it!

Far from it. I would basically have a bowl of cereal in the morning and then starve myself all day until I got home. Then I would proceed to eat everything in sight. My reasoning was that I could work an extra 30 minutes if I didn't stop to eat lunch. This way of eating destroyed my metabolism, meaning I had a very slow metabolism.

The nutritionist gave me an understanding of the problem and a plan to replace my old habit with a new one. I just had to follow the plan. I had to eat more, eat the right things, and eat often, which is counterintuitive to what I'd thought. By the end of my time with the nutritionist I had gone from 19% body fat to just under 10%. With the consistent good eating habits and running three days a week, I got lean. But it took a reversal of a personal "truth" to see the results I wanted.

Listening was a similar insight. I believed I listened well. I could hold a conversation, let others speak, and even pull information out of people. But James C. Petersen's *Why Don't We Listen Better? Communicating and Connecting in Relationships* had new information. This was the gut punch that opened my eyes: "The need-to-win and to put ourselves above others in relationships causes even more problems than shoddy communication."

Through the explanations in this book, I was haunted by how backwards I'd been living. For decades I'd been listening with the intent to get something from others. I would listen and wait until I could show my expertise and knowledge about the way I thought best to handle a situation. I didn't need a friend, nutritionist, or counselor to make it more clear. Once it came into view, it was true.

My listening was self-serving, and it was a reflection of the rest of my life. I was seeing this truth in relationships, where I spent my time, and what I purchased. There was a second layer of understanding that was more true than what I said or felt for the many years I held an alternative view. This tangible layer was the pattern of habit. It was the rubber on the road.

There was nothing I could deny here. Reasons and justifications of why and how I got here didn't matter. I owned how I showed up and treated others. I owned what I was trying to get from life. It wasn't pretty to look at, and this wasn't who I wanted to show up like.

I remember thinking about some of this information. For example, "Listening plus anything wasn't listening." It made my excuses weak and the truth of that was unbreakable. In most of my life I would add to everything I was hearing to get what I wanted, and that was to control the outcome.

I remember talking to my wife as I was reading. I confessed about how I approached our relationship and how I would only listen so that I could show a better way of doing something. Really to show my value. It covered my insecurity and fears.

I was so focused on my issues, I wasn't considering her or anyone else. In doing this, I subconsciously was telling her that she had little value, insinuating she was less than human. On some level I'd known I wasn't really listening, but I hadn't known how it was affecting those around me.

In essence, I was telling her that I didn't believe she could come up with the right answer and I needed to make the right answer known without saying it. This pattern had to be slowly disconnecting us. How frustrating it must have been to be told an answer when you weren't asking for it. How fortunate it was to see this wrong and have time to make it right.

I thought that I had been listening, but really I was asking her opinion and then holding a long enough conversation to refute every aspect that didn't agree with my own opinion. I wasn't truly considering her or her ideas.

Really, there was little intent to take her side. I was mostly out to make sure that our decisions came out the way I thought they should. Not that I only cared about what I wanted, but the results had to come in the way I thought they should, which was the "best" way. Somehow I assumed that only I could see into the future, and my dreamt-up reality was the one that was best. That wasn't even close to the truth.

Like most couples starting out, finances can make a relationship difficult. I remember arguing over purchases and budgets. Never really that heated, but we weren't on the same page. I was always trying to work things the way I believed was right for us. She might remember it differently.

It was a seesaw battle for a while as we tried different ways to structure how to make decisions. I mentioned that my wife manages our family and household. Looking back on the situation, I used to fight to maintain control over finances.

Then it dawned on me, if in running my painting business I was always asked to give validation or had to request approval, it would be awful. But this was what was happening for my wife. I wasn't trusting her to make a good decision. I believed that I needed to be involved to make sure it worked out. The insights from the truth about how I wasn't really listening revealed a depth well beyond what I could pick up at first. The more time I spent tracing back the symptoms to the cause, the more clearly I could recognize when I was "not listening" and, instead, pursuing what I thought was best.

She was patient, we both had a lot to figure out, but I was still immature.

What was comical is that I really just never knew what I wanted out of life, yet I was telling others—in this case my wife and our family—what to do with theirs.

So I changed. She didn't need me to make decisions for us. We chose to give her the majority of the responsibility over our financial decisions. It was hers to do with what she needed. And you know what? It's worked out quite fine without me.

SCENIC OVERLOOK

- Typically, there is a major disconnect between what we think is true versus reality.
- To bridge this disconnect, we can observe—i.e., take an inventory on—what is true (versus what we wish to be true).
- Part of observing is consulting with outside sources that will inform and challenge us to open our typically limited and biased take on the world.

PERSONAL DECLINATION

- Take a little time and think about a long-time frustration or recurring problem you've had. Feel free to write out what you see.
- How would you summarize your observations?
- What are some assumptions you make?
- How have you contributed to your own frustration, regardless of it being your fault or not?
- How would you advise a friend to address this?
- From this exercise, what has changed about how you view the frustration?

OUT-AND-BACK EXERCISE

During the day or week, take the frustration or problem from above (or another example) and apply a change to it. Try not to worry about the results, and focus on trying a new way to approach a familiar problem.

- Write down what you observed as a result of the change. This could be a result or how you felt about the situation.

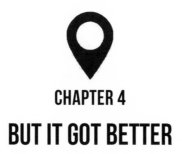

CHAPTER 4

BUT IT GOT BETTER

"When you're looking at the world from a place of misunderstanding, the goals you come up with will reflect that misunderstanding. When you're looking at the world from a place of clarity, the goals you come up with will reflect that clarity."

— *The Little Book of Results:*
A Quick Guide to Achieving Big Goals
by Jamie Smart

This final chapter on my backstory shows how insights I gained in my quest for a new way to approach life began to shape the framework of Compass Form. As these insights are uncovered you'll see how these changes impacted the results. You'll notice how my adjusted perspective helped build my confidence to engage with my story at a greater level. That's the goal for you too: to be able to apply Compass Form, so you can engage with your story at a greater level.

SLIVER OF HOPE

These small changes kept adding up in my relationship with my wife. Fortunately, we both had great examples of marriage from our parents. This was a benefit early on. My wife is really special. She is a supporter and a peacemaker, and I'd say that contributed to the lack of colossal disruptions in our first years of marriage.

But she was noticing the changes happening in my life, and the marriage went from good to even better. Our direction shifted from growing apart to joining together. We began aligning goals. And the results in my life were starting to show up in her life as well.

Consistency was building. Paint, home, read, sleep, and a slow process of growth to move away from the old habits to the new. As the family life was maturing, the painting company was following. On one hand, there was a change and new path to follow. On the other, I was still stuck with work that kept stealing a little more happiness from my (then) dwindling cup of joy.

It's a funny juxtaposition when life becomes more simple and easy, but the level of hope diminishes. Success was finally coming. Jobs were coming in without me going out and finding new work. Around year five, I never had to market for work again. I stopped all advertising and slowly began to increase the profit for my labor. Because I never wanted to have employees, the only way to increase what I took home was to decrease expenses.

I was starting to practice a new approach to life with the space the efficiency of my business created. I began observing my life from an outside perspective now that I had time to slow my mind. What I found is that I love working for people. I really enjoy helping people get to where they want to go. I really like listening. I actually love listening. And I'm talking real, sincere, no-strings-attached listening.

I could get an estimate done in about ten minutes, but around that time estimates started taking over an hour. Why? Because I liked to hear what people were about and I'd ask questions and it led somewhere unexpected.

I had no agenda on estimates, I knew the job was there to be had, and I knew that as long as I didn't lose trust, I'd get the work. So I didn't need to carry the tension of how the arrangement would work out. I was free to be present with strangers and hear them. I could hear concerns and help them address the challenges with hiring a painter. But conversations became about more than painting.

I've had estimates that took over three hours. I've been at a site for eight hours and only worked an hour of it as I've listened to clients share their challenges and perspectives. I would get lost in deep and meaningful conversations with random people. We now have family friends that started from these conversations.

In this way I cut my teeth with coaching well before I ever got certified. Being an introvert, I can't stand chitchat. I loathe small group settings, especially with random strangers. It's overwhelming because I want to figure out what is going on and there is too much to take in. But when I am talking one-on-one and can focus on one thing at a time, I take a conversation deep and quickly. Because I have spent so many hours observing how my internal process works, I imagine how other people process and think, and use that to help guide them to their own answers, using a similar model from my own life.

I found that there are layers to peel back in my life and others have similar layers. Frustrations are the response to results or outcomes. Outcomes are the results of habits. Habits are the growth of desire. And desire shows me what direction I am looking in and heading.

Where I am heading shows me what I believe to be true. And this is true for every individual. To say it in different words: your results, whether good or bad or something in between, all stem from your individual truths, even if you aren't cognizant of this foundational connection.

CUTTING THE ROPE

I mentioned earlier that I jokingly classify myself as a "high functioning, but severely introverted" person. I communicate out of necessity and purpose. Talking with strangers sucks energy from me, and I get tired being in new group conversations.

Mostly the draining comes from anxiety or not understanding how a new situation works. Under that anxiety is fear. But I can't live life without communicating. Previously my communication was limited to getting what I wanted. It was a minimal approach to avoiding the loss of energy.

Growing a business, a coaching practice was impossible if my goal was to avoid people. I was facing the decision that summarizes a lot of what I've been talking about, and that is when you are calm enough to **observe** your circumstance, the most pertinent issue will show up with a little **focus**.

Once you find the **source of the dilemma** and **lostness**, you can address it. The source of the dilemma that arose for me after I did some observing and focusing was this: I could either stay introverted, which would really make building a coaching practice challenging; or I could find a way to set out and meet people, so I could share my passion to help others find their direction, which, in turn, would likely grant me the satisfying career that I had long been craving.

I couldn't do both. They were in stark contrast. North and south. One way would take me in the opposite direction of the other.

I had to commit to one. I couldn't say yes and then turn around. I think a lot of my **life was spent in cycles** like this, but I never saw it clearly (no observation). Therefore, I **got stuck** a lot. **I was stuck in the middle of a decision, and I didn't want to choose.** But the choice was clear now. I could stay as I was and avoid others. Or I could leave comfort to begin a new approach and engage the world around me. Both choices came at a cost. For the longest time leaving my comfort had been a much higher cost. I was learning how to focus on what to do next and not worry about the cost.

This wasn't an easy decision. But it was a simple one. And I chose to change. I had been stuck for so long, it seemed like the only option left. My way wasn't working, and I had to "lose" at that. Losing perceived safety was the cost.

So I left safety and the fear that kept me tied down and set out into the unknown. I have an old pastor friend that I would meet up with and he would ask me this question, "What is keeping you tied to the dock?" Most of the time I would nod and awkwardly smile because not only did I not have an answer, I didn't understand what he meant.

Now I understood, and I knew the answer: fear of the unknown was the rope around me.

That day I learned how to look at a problem and choose to **act** based on the direction that aligned best with what I knew I needed to do. Whether I was scared or not wasn't helpful or even valid. It didn't matter anymore. If I was to go after the direction of my passion, my fear was useless to inform me on the right way to go.

I chose to become a coach at that moment. To be specific, I chose to help people connect with their life in the way I just had. I chose to leave a life that was flat and lifeless to chase a life that was full and significant.

Here is the best part. It was at that moment that I found an even bigger treasure.

It made the pain and suffering of the past redemptive. It made the years before I was able to break away from painting palatable. It made what ended up being a 12-year journey worthwhile. I needed to struggle this long in order to get to this answer. The continued call back to the same problem revealed this hidden secret.

The pain was now worth the cost. The decade-plus of frustration to find answers that I had been railing against for so long was now a savior. It trained me to see a world in a deeper manner than success would have.

I wanted to and would have quit many times before. I attempted to get out in so many different ways and for such a long time. I think if I'd gotten my way, getting out of the painting business too early would have destroyed me. But when the right time came, my eyes were opened to this story loop. I had learned how to push past the panic of not knowing. To see that there was a bigger story in play for me that I hadn't been aware of.

COMPASS FORM'S FOUNDATION

So this is the foundation:

- The moments of life are always bigger than they appear.
- The tragedy is worth the redemption.

- The bigger world isn't out to get me or you, and we can trust that there is always more than our finite perspective.
- Each of us really doesn't have much control or choice.
- If we want to pursue our passion, we have to take that focus and find a way to act on it in every decision.

How we feel might show us a few things about a situation, but it is the wrong conversation to have as often it is useless data that comes from a similar but unrelated past situation. The conversation we need to have with ourselves is: "If this is the direction that I need to go, what is one way that I can get a little closer?"

It didn't make sense to walk in a thousand directions, to head up the mountain and then walk back down and try another trail. We have to push through the unknown of the trail if we want to get to the end of it.

COMPASS FORM

In 2017, I made the decision to pursue coaching as a career. To invest in a program to try and get out of the painting business and push myself further into that unknown direction. The more I invested time, energy, and money, the more I would see a tighter focus for my own direction grow and corresponding results. That ended up leading me to figure out a way to get out. Finally.

I started with offering up coaching for free. Mostly friends, but eventually I started to find some paying clients, and those clients started to see results. I had people almost doubling their incomes as a result of our sessions together. I had people fixing their marriages without even intending to. I had clients enjoying their lives in new ways they weren't considering. It seemed random, or so I thought.

So I took what was common in the thousands of conversations and distilled them into a simple framework—Compass Form—I now use to guide clients to **navigate uncertainty between where someone is and the big and small ideas they want to get to.** What I love about this framework is that it isn't meant to restrain you. There is nothing to keep in mind and adhere to. You are fine to live your life, and if you get stuck or lost, then this tool will help you find your way.

Compass Form is meant to be adaptable. It is meant to be put away when it isn't needed, so that you can be in full experience of what is going on, in the now, and make decisions based on where you aim to go. This is similar to holding an actual compass in that you'll miss out on life if you are always staring down at the tool.

One of the problems I have had with most trainings and self-help systems is that you are taking someone else's journey and trying to make it yours. I found myself wanting to closely model the success I saw in others. I wanted help to get to where I thought I needed to go, to learn another skill so that I could "start" the next project. But help never came. I invested in expensive programs and free courses. The result was always the same. The outcome never looked as good as the sales pitch, and I never saw the same results that were promised.

After a while I began to take inventory on what was the common challenge for me after working through a course or training. I noticed that my story was never the same as the person leading the group or the others in the group. I found myself looking to mirror the results of someone else rather than being mindful of my own journey.

So I would be looking at what someone else was telling me to do and not spending time on what I should be doing. And that was a problem. The truth is, I am the only person who can write the story of my life. You are the only person who can write the story of your life.

Another big point was that when I started a course, I approached my circumstances very differently than when I initially signed up for it. Some courses were one week and some were six months. But I noticed that my life was never the same, week to week, even day to day. Most every course I took was teaching a process that was not permeable and adaptable. Their plan was stagnant, but my life changed so quickly, it couldn't keep up. That was a problem.

The final lesson was that I was left to try and figure out if I was doing the process right. I was again focused on the coursework and learning, and not on my own situation. I was uncertain because I was starting out and when the results didn't come, I was attributing that to having done something wrong, missing a step. That was leaving me anxious and hesitant to move ahead. That was a problem.

So I needed a way to deal with these major problems, and I knew that in working with others, they did as well. What came about was the framework I call Compass Form. The framework addresses each of these problems and also provides a simple way for you to clearly understand where you are, where you want to go, and what you can do to get there.

I needed Compass Form to be **flexible**. I needed it to be **universal**. I needed it to be **simple**. Life gives us enough to carry and keep track of. I wasn't interested in adding more and spending all my time learning a system. I assumed no one else wanted to either.

When someone else tried to write my story for me, the plans and processes were isolated in nature. They were contingent on dominating other areas of my life. They were poised as silver bullets but couldn't even fix the original problem I was having. They created chaos and not simplicity.

This framework is meant **to give life back and not take from it.** It's a simple way to see through to your life because the challenges that you have and will face are real and not easy. It creates a way for you—and anyone—to get through the tragedies and set a course to follow the direction you need to go, no matter how challenging the journey is to get there.

So I created Compass Form, three simple steps that you can adapt to any situation at any point in time. I looked back on the success of the people I was working with and the success I had seen with my own life and summarized them into Compass Form's observe, focus, and act.

SCENIC OVERLOOK

- When you are calm enough to observe your true circumstance (as opposed to your biased perception of it), the ideal area for you to address will show up with a little focus.
- Once you find the source of the dilemma and lostness, you can address it.
- Compass Form is a flexible, universal, and simple framework for navigating uncertainty.
- Compass Form gives life back to you.

PERSONAL DECLINATION

- What are you recognizing in your own life as you read through the first few chapters?
- What truth is becoming apparent for you, even if it isn't yet fully formed and easy to articulate?
- How would you feel if you moved beyond what has been holding you back?
- What is an area that you have interest in pursuing?
- What is a simple change that you could try?

OUT-AND-BACK EXERCISE

Focus on an area you want to change. Let go of the results and outcomes for the moment.

- What are a few ways to approach what you'd like to change in a new way? What could make even the slightest impact on what you'd like to see happen?

It's worth noting that "right" doesn't matter and isn't the focus of the exercise. It's more important that you can consider a change that might not seem like the best idea at first glance.

- How did your expectations change in letting go of a predetermined outcome to get it "right"?

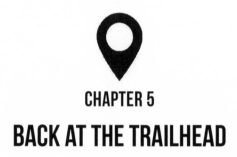

CHAPTER 5

BACK AT THE TRAILHEAD

"Many people think they lack motivation when what they really lack is clarity. It is not always obvious when and where to take action. Some people spend their entire lives waiting for the time to be right to make an improvement."

—*Atomic Habits: An Easy and Proven Way to Build Good Habits and Break Bad Ones*
by James Clear

In order to best understand how effective Compass Form is in allowing you to make progress and move forward in your life, in this chapter we will explore Compass Form as it generally works. How exactly you will learn and apply it comes in a later chapter. To best grasp the beauty of Compass Form we'll start exploring it by comparing it to the typical perspective that most of us take in approaching life. This typical perspective is one that most often leads to us being stuck or moving in circles. In chapters 2 to 4 you saw already many of these characteristics of the "stuck" perspective as they played out in my life before I realized Compass Form. We are reviewing them briefly again in this chapter because the better you can recognize them for how stealthily and powerfully disruptive they are, then the more you'll recognize the beauty of Compass Form as a way to correct and/or avoid the problems the "stuck" perspective brings.

RUNNING A RACE VS. CAPTAINING A SHIP

Most people tend to have one of two perspectives when it comes to engaging life. The first is the running-a-race perspective. People who live from this perspective approach their lives similarly to someone who is running a race. The runner has a determined course to run that has an apparent start and finish. The goal of the runner is to precisely follow the given course and finish the race as quickly as possible in order to win. The perspective that a runner takes is to be efficient with running and to maximize how quickly the course can be traveled, as the route won't change and it is simply a matter of time to complete the route. The runner is looking for the most effective way to run, and delays or obstacles are hindrances that are unexpected.

The second perspective is like a captain of a ship in that while a captain might have a determined end, the route they take is all the time being adjusted due to the ever-changing current, wind, and weather conditions. The goal of the captain is to be ready for changes and adjust the course as needed. The captain is anticipating the route to change and is looking to stay on course by using tools to discover how much the course has moved. The captain is on the lookout for obstacles and ready to apply skills to adjust for them. While there's an ultimate destination, the journey itself is not prescribed, so problems are expected. As I expect you already realized, Compass Form promotes the captaining a ship approach to life.

So many people engage with their lives from the perspective of running a race. They just want to get to the finish of the current goal or get out of a bad situation. But there is a downside to the running-a-race perspective in that people who engage the world in this manner are repeatedly shocked that life isn't a clean race to run (even though they "know it" on some level). They are continually frustrated that there always seems to be a problem that gets in the way of the race. They get upset because each new obstacle surprises them. They are annoyed and dismayed when they are forced to pivot in order to get around challenges.

It is understandable that people with the running-a-race perspective get upset because they are working very hard to run as fast as they can and when a change of course comes, they do not have the extra energy (or the spirit) to pivot with because they didn't anticipate the additional work. Most of us are exhausted from the amount of effort we use to get to the finish. Real-life obstacles could include not getting the raise we deserve, unexpected expenses, untimely and surprising injuries, how much time and energy it takes to raise children, losing a parent too soon, or an unexpected weather condition that interrupts traffic.

What I am not saying is that this perspective is wrong or ignorant. What I am saying is that the running-a-race perspective leaves us at the mercy of the idea of what things (supposedly) should look like when we started the race. The runner has a fixed picture of the race, and any shift is looked at as a problem that should not have happened. This perspective hinders us from expediently handling problems that arise because we react to the pain of the problem (rather than handling the problem itself) and allow that pain to incapacitate us.

The captain's perspective cares less for the road map to look the same as it did when the journey started. A captain doesn't exactly have a map. Instead, a captain has a general direction. They've already learned to use tools to help them identify where they are at, to respond to a wide range of troubling conditions, and to regain course to eventually reach their final destination.

Let's take a look at how these approaches might play out in real life. Say, for instance, how people approach going to the grocery store. It's a simple example that can usually translate to more complex situations seeing as most of us use the same techniques for easy and complex scenarios.

A person with the running-a-race perspective would probably approach grocery shopping like a race. They know success is getting through the store as quickly as possible, with everything they need in the store in its designated spot, and people working every register, so lines move quickly. When any of the planned parts of the grocery shopping become disrupted, the "runner" person gets thrown out of balance emotionally, becoming frustrated, impatient, and maybe even aggressive.

In contrast, a captain perspective would anticipate that even though they are hoping to avoid disruptions while grocery shopping, more than likely this will not be the case, so they prepare accordingly. They might leave a few minutes early to give themselves a time cushion, and they don't take out their frustrations on employees, other customers, or other vehicles on the road.

Again, there is no judgment to say which perspective is better or worse, but something to note is that neither perspective influences whether and how many obstacles a person encounters. Instead, both perspectives influence the mental, emotional, and energy states of the person holding them. I'll add that it is amazing that with the running-a-race perspective, we tend to not anticipate disruptions to how we think the journey should go.

Comparing these two perspectives points to a major difference that most of us don't pick up on. We live a lot of life with a mental idea of what life should be, so much so that often we are not aware of what is going on in real life around us because we're so caught up in notions in our mind. When that happens, our view of the world narrows and we become less capable of adaptation to the real world around us. We get to where we must have the world work out in a specific way for it to seem "right" to us.

With the running-a-race perspective we are looking for the external world to live up to what we envision on the inside, in our mind. And when that doesn't happen, we grow frustrated, we tend to panic or feel anxious, and we might even get angry. With the captain's perspective, we are more focused on observing the internal temperature of our lives because we know the external is changing, so more often than not, we will need to adjust accordingly.

At this point, you are hopefully recognizing the way you approach the world and the perspective you most often carry. It is even easier to see when we are stressed out. By default we revert to what seems easier to us. There are many more perspectives that people have, but generally speaking these two are pretty good summaries of where all perspectives end up falling in relationship to each other. So the real challenge that should be presenting itself is that those of us who approach life with the running-a-race perspective, in fact, should not be surprised that we become upset when life changes around us.

RUNNING A RACE	CAPTAINING A SHIP
The Approach to Life That Often Results In Stagnancy and Dissatisfaction	Compass Form—The Flexible Approach That Allows Us to Expediently Respond to Real Life As It Happens
• Narrowing your focus too closely on the end goal and the prescribed, anticipated steps to reach it • Allowing your feelings to determine success or failure • Worrying about a choice being right or wrong • Allowing any obstacles to cause a quitting mentality • Avoiding changing course • Comparing to others' success	• Holding, at most moments, an awareness of the ultimate destination but cognizant of the fact there are no exact, must-have, prescribed steps to reach it • Noticing feelings and using them to show you what can be changed • Focusing on what is effective effort • Allowing obstacles to show you new opportunities • Anticipating how to adjust to stay on course • Trusting that you will find a way • Looking to stay aware of the next step to take regardless of the outlook

A FEW MORE SCENARIOS

As already noted, this chapter's aim is for you to gain a big picture grasp of Compass Form. This brings us to the next step. Here, we'll look at some example scenarios that involve more comparing and contrasting so that you can gain a strong understanding of Compass Form.

SCENARIO 1—TRYING TO LOSE WEIGHT RUNNING-A-RACE APPROACH

Let's revisit this example I gave in an earlier chapter when I wanted to lose weight. As I already wrote, I was gaining weight and didn't want it to continue. I had been running for a few years, but it wasn't enough to keep me from adding on pounds. How I'd been eating for so many years was like this: I would basically have a bowl of cereal in the morning and then starve myself all day until I got home. Then I would proceed to eat everything in sight. My reasoning is that I could work an extra 30 minutes if I didn't stop to eat lunch.

Why was my original way of eating like the running-a-race approach? Because I wasn't looking to solve the problem. The goal was to lose weight, but I wasn't giving much thought as to what the cause of the weight gain was. After a small breakfast, I assumed it was fine to gorge in the evening because I hadn't eaten all day. I assumed that my eating was fine. This was an illusion, reality didn't match. I was reacting to what I thought was true from my past experience, rather than observing what was potentially contributing to gaining weight. What I was really trying to do was put in minimal effort and hope that it would be enough. I didn't want to stop and take a good look at things. This is similar to running a race by focusing on getting around the obstacle as quickly as possible rather than getting real and addressing the obstacle and then correcting course.

CAPTAINING A SHIP—COMPASS FORM APPROACH

When I started working with a nutritionist, the nutritionist gave me an understanding of the problem and a plan to replace my old habit with a new one. I had to eat more, eat the right things, and eat often. By the end of my time with the nutritionist I had gone from 19% body fat to just under 10%. With the consistent good eating habits and running, I got lean.

Why is this like captaining a ship? Because I got out of my head and didn't rely on my assumptions about how reality (in this case, my metabolism) worked. I looked to get ahead of the problem. I got out of my head by consulting with an expert who is trained in the area (and discontinued living on imagined beliefs as I had been doing). Because I acted on the intention, I found out something new and was able to change the course to how I wanted to show up in life. I had the best information to work from. Once I observed the true problem, adjusting course was simple. Not to say it was easy because change still comes at a cost. But instead of trying to figure out what to do and also fighting to change my lifestyle, I was able to simply focus on sticking to the new eating plan. Since I had taken the time to build the intention, I had an intention to fall back on. Working on one challenge at a time was paramount to following through and getting to where I wanted to go.

SCENARIO 2—FINDING A NEW JOB
RUNNING-A-RACE APPROACH

A common struggle I've run into with clients is around work and finding a job or career they would enjoy. When someone wants to change their job, they typically start searching job sites for work that lines up with their experience. Finding the new job becomes the race. They look for a job that fits their skills and pays a little more than their current one. When they finally find the position that lines up in their mind, they might run through a pro and con list of past data and chat with a few friends about it. They try and find the perfect fit, but usually settle for any change of work. They become skilled at using a process to switch jobs. But in a few years or even months, the shine wears off and they start considering jumping again. It is becoming a cycle now. Most people with this perspective aren't looking at what is causing job dissatisfaction; instead, they are focused on switching jobs.

This is similar to the runner putting all their effort into crossing the finish line at the expense of the whole journey: "Don't like my job. Find a new job." The assumption is that whatever is missing or dissatisfying about the current job can be found in a new one. Attention isn't given to the cause of dissatisfaction, and quickly running around that obstacle (and never addressing it) is what happens. Once the idea is set in their mind, the focus is only on finding the next job. The reality of that new job and any obstacles that might come with it—and whether or not it truly suits them and will be satisfying to them—isn't something they consider. It's all about the end goal, a new job.

CAPTAINING A SHIP—COMPASS FORM APPROACH

Using Compass Form for job searching might look like this. Through observation look at what is broken with the current situation. But also look at what you believe would make any job enjoyable or not. Consider what is meaningful in this position and in previous jobs to see if any patterns show up. That way when it comes time to consider whether to stay or leave a position you have an accurate account of what to ask yourself and others when considering changing.

Question yourself as to why a new job will make your life better. It would involve taking inventory on where the gaps are from what the current job provides to what your ideal work would look like. It would pause to see if there are ways to change the current situation. It would look past the job to understand what the real goal of your work would be. It would expand the focus of finding a job. There would be consideration of multiple ways to experience enjoyment from work. End goal is to know what is causing the desire to change before making a change.

SCENARIO 3—A FALTERING MARRIAGE RUNNING-A-RACE APPROACH

Here, let's look at a marriage that after five years becomes unbearable. There have been good days but a lot of bad days. Eventually the attempts to make a good marriage wear away. Rather than trying to make things work, one spouse becomes convinced that they married the wrong person because of the amount of pain they experience. There isn't much thought given to what a good marriage is only that they want what a good marriage "should be." Please note, this topic is by far much more complex, and no justice is done by simplifying the specifics of any relationship.

With the running-a-race approach, a person assumes that a marriage should default to good, and they experience shock and disappointment when the relationship doesn't effortlessly, automatically play out that way. The runner-type person doesn't anticipate problems to come and blames their spouse when problems arise. Divorce ultimately becomes the new finish line that will solve everything because the runner person believes they can leave the broken pieces of the "bad" marriage behind and try afresh, this time with the "right" person. In the end, the idea is that swapping out one person for another will relieve the distress and solve the problem of the "bad" marriage.

What happens is the person is applying their old habits that created problems in one relationship into another. More than likely the second relationship will eventually mirror the first.

CAPTAINING A SHIP—COMPASS FORM APPROACH

To approach a faltering marriage using Compass Form, we would start by observing the tension in a relationship with the aim of identifying the true source(s). Without changing the influence and inputs that create the separation in the relationship, it would be unwise to believe problems will not continue. Since the goal is to build a well-functioning relationship, the focus spotlights effective changes and preparing for unseen problems. A relationship is never on cruise control and adjustments are a must. Empathy is found in that both people understand that each is not perfect. Patience is given to navigate life together. A captain anticipates having to throw needed cargo overboard to lighten the load and navigate shallow waters. This may come at a cost of personal happiness in the short term much like any course adjustment does. There is creativity in solving issues and tension. They eventually can see any "loss of cargo" is insignificant if the ship stays afloat.

SCENARIO 4—A SPORTS OPPORTUNITY RUNNING-A-RACE APPROACH

There is an opportunity for your child to play on a local travel team. Here is what usually floods into someone's head: *How much does it cost? Can I afford that? Will we have time to get the child to practice and when are practices? How long will the season go for? And what about the vacation we are trying to plan? I wonder if this sport could allow them someday to get a college scholarship? Should they even go to college?* You can see how quickly our mind races towards trying to solve many decisions at once. The ideas come quickly like a firehose.

In this scenario, in engaging the running-a-race approach, you would more than likely create a predetermined outcome that you want to see happen: either to join or not join. In conversations with your child you would try and guide them to your way of wanting it to play out. If you want your child to participate, you'd steer them to that decision. Your goal might be to convince them to see it your way. As a result, you might get frustrated if your child isn't enthusiastic or as committed as you are or want them to be. Often these conversations are focused on a short-term sprint. You take the many questions and choices and try to get through them as quickly as possible. Decisions become an overwhelming nuisance because they are distracting you from reaching your bigger goal. People become obstacles. This is like running a race because your focus is on the end—the goal of getting your child to accept what will help you get through these many obstacles as quickly as possible.

CAPTAINING A SHIP—COMPASS FORM APPROACH

A captaining approach would be looking to leverage the sports season as a way to grow a child as a whole. It would be less reactive to disruptions and making sure the timeline was adhered to. Despite being busy there would be time to pause and reflect. Time to adjust approaches. Yours and your child's.

This is like captaining because you are looking at the parenting as the experience rather than a game or even a sports season to get through. Every moment, even disruptions or seeming losses, are opportunities for growth, learning, and even fun. The journey is the goal, not an experience to get beyond.

YOUR STANCE: RUNNER OR CAPTAIN?

Many of us get hung up on the disappointment of life because our mindset typically resembles running a race. When we have a new idea, we immediately want to see it come to fruition. What happens is that every obstacle and problem end up being a hindrance and annoyance that limits the potential of the performance and result of the race. The expectation is that if we run fast and hard enough, we should get past the finish line and find peace and joy.

Often what happens is that in the moment, we change and move the line from the original idea, or the original idea isn't vetted well enough, so we end up jumping into a race that we should not be in. Maybe we even leave a good track for a (supposedly) greener one. But the pattern is the same: find a race, put everything into it (short term), and then find frustration when it doesn't work out. Ultimately that disappointment either gets shouldered by us or the people around us.

We are defeated when we don't see the results of the effort that we put in, and we often lash out at those around us when the results don't line up with our expectations. Even though we care about and maybe feel like they won't run away when we react to them in a negative way. From our evil and chaotic side, we demand that they meet the unknown expectations we have set for the world, but in all honesty our thoughts never even leave our minds, let alone give us a decent plan of execution or realistic chance of success, other than "Be positive," "Stop whining," and "Plow through."

Captaining a ship via Compass Form represents an excellent way to navigate your life. When you are aboard a boat, the water and other elements are always shifting. To captain means you are aware of the need to adjust course and are necessarily attentive to your surroundings. It's not like a race where you'd simply set a path and

go, blindly (and vainly) following the exact path no matter what …
and then getting shocked and rattled when you encounter obstacles.

Like a boat, you are constantly drifting, and in order to head towards
what matters most, you will need to create a framework or discipline
to stay aware and simply adjust course. No captain falls asleep and
wakes up to the shock and horror that their boat has moved. Change
is expected and the captain knows how to stay on course or make
corrections when put off course.

No captain uses their tools of navigation once and then hopes to
never use them again. The captain constantly references them,
knowing that the water the boat is on will pose a problem that can't
be ignored. Often the problems are a gift to help develop better tools
that can be used to make the journey more efficient. Not that the
journey becomes easier, but the ability to take on greater challenges
increases. Compass Form is the tool I am sharing in this book, so you
can journey and take on your journey's challenges more efficiently.

Can you keep going through life using the running-a-race approach?
The fact you are reading this book shows that you want out of
that race because you know it'll make for a dismal, frustrating, and
claustrophobic life. It's time to get out the compass and step into
the boat. It's time to change your approach to Compass Form.

As you begin to consider the perspective of working with the
Compass Form framework, it's time to start looking how it can
affect your lifestyle and engagement. It is important to note that
the goal of *Before You Begin* isn't to condemn how people operate in
the world. It is to provide another way for people to find satisfaction
and success. As you consider what Compass Form is and what it
isn't, the remaining chapters will present how you can adapt the
framework to your own life.

At any point in this book, if you want to explore getting personal guidance in engaging Compass Form in your own life, please contact me—jacob@themountainpassway.com and https://themountainpassway.com.

SCENIC OVERLOOK

- Taking a look at goals before you start making plans allows you to open up additional options.
- Seeing multiple options helps you to consider other tools or ways to tackle a problem.
- Looking at your problem with a wider view brings truth.
- Frustration comes from confusion, disappointment, inaccurate assumptions, and unmet expectations.

PERSONAL DECLINATION

- What are some areas of your life that are stuck in automatic?
- When could this be more problematic than healthy?
- How would you use a captaining approach in these areas?

OUT-AND-BACK EXERCISE

Find a recurring frustration. Determine whether you are running a race or captaining a ship in regard to it. Take a look at some other ways to engage. Focus on a better way to handle the frustration, and try it out the next time it comes about.

- How did the results change from the past approach?

CHAPTER 6

APPLYING COMPASS FORM: OBSERVE

"People often think that the best way to predict the future is by collecting as much data as possible before making a decision. But this is like driving a car looking only at the rearview mirror—because data is only available about the past."

—*How Will You Measure Your Life?*
by Clayton M. Christensen,
James Allworth, and Karen Dillon

We've spent a great deal of time establishing the overall characteristics and philosophy behind Compass Form and contrasting that to the more typical "stagnancy-inducing" approach to life that most of us engage, what I've named the running-a-race approach. Now it is time that we move to the application stage: how to engage Compass Form to transform your life for the better, in the short-, medium-, and long-terms.

Essential to applying Compass Form, as first mentioned in chapter 1, is mastering its three parts: observe, focus, and act. These three parts are about isolating the real issue, so you address it accurately and specifically and all the while clear some of the chaos that comes with trying to make a decision in an already busy, decision-filled day (and life). Observe, focus, and act are not about predicting the future because Compass Form is about living in real time, in the present (as much as that is possible considering the ever-moving nature of the present). Life is ambiguous and chaotic. The skill you are building is learning how to quickly make sense of the chaos and being content with a decision. Observe, focus, and act are about settling on a decision and allowing yourself to adjust your course. Observe, focus, and act should provide you enough clarity, so you can move forward and at the same time should leave enough looseness, so you can adjust course as needed.

In this chapter we look at the first step of Compass Form: observe.

OBSERVE OVERVIEW

When you are grappling with an issue, feeling not at ease about something, feeling impatient and frustrated, or attempting to make a change but repeatedly not being able to achieve it, no matter how hard you try—these are all indicators that it's time to engage Compass Form, starting with its first step: observe.

If you typically approach distressing and uncomfortable situations, people, and feelings from a running-the-race perspective, then your first step in handling it is likely not to simply observe. It's likely you want to do something or say something to try to control the obstacle, but as you'll recall from previous chapters, there is very little in life that we can control. And trying to control outside circumstances is often a nonsensical, tedious burden that has little effect and isn't sustainable.

Instead of aiming to quickly act in an attempt to control an obstacle, Compass Form presents a very different way of first engaging: you will actively observe.

What then does it mean to observe? To observe means to locate the current reality, not the past or future, remembered or imagined reality. You must locate the current reality that is not encumbered by the assumptions, blind spots, biases, hopes, and dreams that you might be inadvertently (or not) placing on the obstacle that, in turn, distorts it.

It's amazing how much we can add to a situation that is not relevant. And why is that? Partially because we don't like what we see, we compare ourselves to others around us, we are tired, we are lost, we are overwhelmed, and we are scared.

Each of these biases and blind spots we carry end up covering a reality, so we cannot make out what is going on. Instead, we allow our distorted and inaccurate notion of reality to give us an out to delay and procrastinate. To stay stagnate. To move in circles without making real progress to the ultimate place of what we really want.

The aim of observing is to find the reality of a situation. Only by pausing and making observations to decipher what is real and true versus what are your own clouded, biased assumptions, can you then put into effect the next steps of Compass Form where you focus to determine the most ideal action to take in the given reality and then you do that action.

Taking the time to see what is real (and not only your deduction and guess) is a major part to allow time for you to move from reaction to intention. Compass Form as a whole through this first step of observation really is a practice of checking back in with what is real rather than allowing yourself to get lost in thinking about what could be real. You can dream about running a marathon, and that might assist, but the work of consistent practice is what gets you there. If left to your thinking and wondering about what-if, I'm not sure it would be enough to accomplish anything.

QUESTIONS TO HELP YOU OBSERVE

When you are addressing a disconnect, a source of conflict, a feeling of stress or discomfort around yourself, another person, a situation, or a decision—big or small—it's time to engage Compass Form starting with step one: observe.

The aim of observing is locating what is accurately and in reality going on amidst the appealing yet often distorted ideas, thoughts, possibilities, and chatter that your mind suggests is real. Essentially, it is pausing to take an inventory in order to locate reality.

Here are some guiding questions to pose to yourself when you realize it's time to pause and observe:

- *What is going on right now?*
- *What am I trying to accomplish?*
- *What else?*
- *What is my responsibility and what is the responsibility of others?*
- *How would I want others to approach a similar situation?*
- *What seems to be causing the problem or issue?*
- *What do my feelings tell me about the circumstance?*
- *How else could I look at this circumstance?*
- *What is missing from the picture of my circumstances?*
- *Is this worth the time and energy, or should I move on?*

- *I'll brainstorm any and all info that comes to mind regarding what I have been thinking about, relevant or not … What doesn't make sense? What clear themes or patterns can I see? Can I organize the brainstorm?*
- *I'll take a deep breath and take one last shot at adding something else.*

Let's look at how observe works for a real person, so you can get a better grasp of it to apply it to your life.

ANDREW + OBSERVE

Andrew had been running an independent financial planner practice, but also had to take on a part-time job working for FedEx. He met with me to learn to grow his business.

When Andrew talked to me about what was going on with his financial planning, as you'll notice, he seemed to be trying everything and getting nowhere. Essentially he was expending a lot of effort spinning his wheels with nothing coming of it. You'll notice that he engaged the running-a-race approach when it came to his business.

This is what Andrew explained to me: he was trying to grow his business by increasing marketing, attending more events, and spending additional time and money to increase the reach of his business to new and potential clients. But he was lacking the time, money, and energy to keep this up. He was frustrated about the great amount of effort he was putting in to grow his business and the lack of results. He believed that if he worked hard enough and met the right people, the practice would grow. But he was running out of steam and being pulled apart by the many responsibilities he faced.

As we talked about what he was currently doing, it became evident that he was always looking towards external factors to change and work out. For example, he was trying to build more contact with clients through newsletters and email. And this wasn't going well. When people are trying to find something outside of themselves to fix their circumstances, they believe that the idea will produce results. They end up disconnecting from their passion and what drove them to invest in their work.

Andrew hadn't considered that there was a learning process to be good at communicating with clients and that it would take time and learning. We all tend to get stuck in this type of cycle. We hope the next idea will be the one that makes life easy. Even simple steps take time to implement and master. Reality was that Andrew wanted to change but was only changing the ideas in his mind. He ended up trying out an idea and then quickly moved on to another idea before the original idea had time to mature.

There were a lot of things that he would start and not complete. Part of this comes from having a lot on his plate. He would pick something up to try and fix it and then pick up something else because the first item was difficult or boring. For example, financial planners have a lot of paperwork to work through and file. This was a task that was a challenge for Andrew to complete each week because it didn't make him money. It is a sunk cost that comes with the business.

There were a bunch of random tasks that all took time and added to the complexity of change. Andrew would worry and stress himself in circles with the questions: *What to work on? What results will I get? Is it going to be done right? Will it be worth it?* He started questioning everything, and it played havoc on his confidence and peace of mind.

Boredom with paperwork led him to thinking about gaining clients, which led to the problem of how to find more. This led to worry about never finding them, which showed the concern that he'd be stuck in this situation forever, or even worse, have to go work for someone else to make ends meet. And what if he couldn't find that and maybe loses a client or two? Then he would probably have to sell the house and move in with his in-laws. And how could he be a financial planner if he couldn't manage his own finances?

By asking Andrew the probing "observe" questions and guiding him to be able to ask himself these questions, Andrew was able to sort through the distractions and land on the real issue. His problem wasn't paperwork or landing the next "right" thing to do for his business; his problem was fear. And that fear created panic and a desire to find something outside of himself to fix the fear.

So it seemed that Andrew was running a race and running out of energy to keep going. Fear was getting bigger and more dangerous. Life was becoming burdensome and irritating. And the irritation showed up in meetings with clients and at home with his family. The burdens and being lost keep us from seeing a situation for what it is. We start creating a fiction (rather than recognizing the truth) and try to manage a narrative that isn't real. This is what was happening for Andrew.

As we continued to talk, another reality emerged. It became clear too that Andrew couldn't see or recognize why people worked with him. He thought his value came from working hard and out valuing the competition. He spent so much time thinking about what he wanted for his clients that he missed the obvious patterns that his current clients could provide and he missed connecting with his clients with what they wanted from a financial planner.

Andrew and I began talking about why he got into planning. We talked about what was important for him to provide for his family. He shared an amazing story about working as a life insurance agent before becoming a financial planner. He had some clients that were just starting out in their life together. Unfortunately they experienced a great loss. The husband passed away unexpectedly. This newly married couple were abruptly torn apart, but they had planned in advance with insurance.

Andrew had to provide that check to the widow. And she had no idea what to do with it. She had no plan to use the funds for her benefit. She had a lump sum of cash and no idea where it should go. It was at that moment Andrew picked up on his why. He wanted to help people manage their money well to give them a sense of security. He spent the next five years building a business to do so. But never reflected to see this important truth.

We later discussed what the motivation or outcome was that he was hoping to give to his family. He wanted to provide financially for his family, but did he see how that could be accomplished?

Typically when I coach someone, after observing, I compile and state back to them what I am seeing. In this case, I told Andrew that I observed that he wanted to grow the business. The growth would allow him to quit the part-time job and have more free time to spend with his family and continue to grow the business. He was trying many ideas that never really panned out and after five years was lost as to where to go next. He wanted advice to grow the business and thought that change would fix the problems of his life. While Andrew pursued many fixes, he neglected to recognize the biggest issue: his fear of failing. Also he'd become so distracted by his worries and pursuit of fixes that he'd lost touch with his main driver for getting into financial planning: helping people find security.

In the coming chapters on focus and act, we will return to Andrew to notice how those phases of Compass Form played out for him. As of right now, the important takeaway is to notice how Andrew distorted reality and how my guiding Andrew to engage with the observe step helped him to locate what was true and accurate versus what wasn't.

A DEEP BREATH AND A SECOND LOOK

When you think back to two issues that I outlined about myself earlier in the book—my struggle to lose weight and my lack of real listening—it was only by pausing and observing that I was able to locate the predominant issue that was keeping me from success. In terms of losing weight, I engaged a nutritionist who clued me in on the reality of how the metabolism worked. In terms of listening, I read a book that clued me in on the true nature of listening. From there, I asked myself, "What is going on in real time when I'm supposedly listening to others?" to realize that I tended to appear to be listening while, in fact, I was waiting to assert my agenda. In both these situations it was pausing to observe and locate reality that enabled me to move toward real progress and change.

While the result of observing may be an "AHA!" moment, it could also be much more nuanced than that. For example, a release of tension or a subtle shift that you might barely notice or only notice upon later reflection.

I was talking with a friend the other day about a potential living situation change he was going to have to make. His current rental was being sold, and there was no option to stay. As he talked through the scenario and his attempts to find a new place to live, it came to his mind that to move to a new location might actually require a major lifestyle change. One of the changes would be no off-street parking.

It was during this conversation we observed that he currently greatly valued doing mechanic-type work on a vehicle. However, that wouldn't be possible if he only had street parking. While it would be simple and normal to spend extra on storing a second vehicle somewhere to maintain his current way of life, it might actually be more of a pain to bring his tools and workshop with him to a storage location. Plus, his life in the near future wouldn't be as flexible to allow him the time and energy to keep with it. While it wasn't fun for him to consider that he'd have to give up this beloved activity, he found it valuable to think about and acknowledge how greatly his mechanic-type work mattered to him. Something he hadn't totally realized before.

Notice by observing, my friend's agenda in speaking to me shifted from finding a place to live to what was really at play in his heart: acknowledging how important his mechanic work was to him and how in moving, he'd likely have to begin a new phase of life without this work that's brought him so much satisfaction. When there is time to pause and look at our reality, personal truths and additional possibilities come up. A new conversation begins that will allow us to create a better understanding of what matters right now and what needs to be looked at more deeply. While there is still a chance that my friend can continue his interest, the change of lifestyle will cost him something different in the future. By acknowledging all of this, my friend puts himself in a better position to seek out a solution or make other adjustments to contend with what matters greatly to him.

To repeat: observe is about recognizing where you are right now, not where you'd like to be, or where you think you should be, but a realistic look at what is going on right now. Once you have begun to observe, you can start to focus, which is narrowing down to the single issue you want to address. And this second step—"focus"—is the focus of the next chapter.

SCENIC OVERLOOK

- Observe is giving yourself a chance to pause and consider what is true.
- Observe widens your point of view.
- Observe defines the problem or goal holistically.
- Observe reduces past and future biases.
- Observe allows you to find causes for the symptoms.

PERSONAL DECLINATION

- What was significant about the observation phase?
- What observations did you make about your own circumstances while reading this chapter?
- What might keep you from taking the time to observe—to look more intently at—your frustration or goal?
- How can you avoid staying in the loop of observing?

OUT-AND-BACK EXERCISE

Go to a public space or grab coffee with a friend with the intention of observing people around you. Set in your mind before heading out to observe only. Observe and not analyze. Just notice. Give yourself a few minutes to watch what is going on. Don't be creepy either.

- What did you see?
- What observations did you take away from the situation?
- How did not being directly impacted from the scenario change how you took in information?

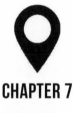

CHAPTER 7

APPLYING COMPASS FORM: FOCUS

"When following a bearing, it is best to find some object, such as a big rock or a unique-looking tree, that is in the same direction as the desired bearing. Then put the compass away and walk toward that object until you arrive at it, and repeat the process with another visible landmark. This is far better (safer and faster) than walking along, compass in hand, constantly observing the compass, rather than watching where you are going."

—*Wilderness Navigation*
by Bob Burns and Mike Burns

At the end of the last chapter, I shared a story about a friend who was in the process of moving from a rental. Note the shift in the conversation from finding a place to live to considering a new way to live. This is the transitioning process of focus. The end of observing is the beginning of focus. For my friend, the shift opened up the true nature of what moving might mean for him and how he wanted to show up in the future. When we focus, there is a narrowing in on a course that makes good sense. This happens naturally, and as clarity emerges, we are pulled into resolving the true nature of our problems.

FOCUS OVERVIEW

Observe might be the easiest to enact, and focus might be the most difficult. Especially when you first begin to use Compass Form, you may spend more time observing than is necessary. As you become more comfortable with the process, you'll see that your thinking speeds up dramatically almost to the place that you are forgetting that you are observing, and you seem to jump straight to focus. As this happens, you are forgoing the need to create a fictional story and homing in on what is going on.

Focus solves the dilemma of getting stuck in observing and not making meaningful changes in your life. When you focus, you take the questions of observe, such as "Where am I now?" and "What is available to me?" and look for a response and action to take from what you learned about your situation or yourself. Focus means you ask, "So what? What do I want to do about what I just observed?" or "What exactly do I want to work towards now that I have uncovered something new and relevant to my life?"

Focus helps you to quickly identify your values and determine the opportunities that line up with those values. How you feel—stressed, annoyed, worried, hurt, afraid—drops in priority and gives way to you finding something meaningful to work towards, a focus for yourself.

How you feel won't matter if you move towards what is most important to you. Focus is not taking a step of action, but it clarifies your heart and core. If you aren't excited or sure of what you decide to focus on, then it is probably not what you are looking for. It's not connected to one of your core values.

There is no alternative for you to see what is important to you. There is no way to gain a brighter clarification anywhere else on

JACOB COLDWELL

the planet. You are the best captain of your ship. Even in your least mature states, you can hear the heart and core (soul) of your being and notice how your observations align with it. This will lead to you narrowing down to what is important and what to "focus" on.

Focus identifies how to align the opportunities that are coming. It is a necessary self-judgement to run your options through and a decision-maker to give basis and reasoning to eliminate one choice or continue with another. Focus is made in real time and isn't held up by the past or the future. It sits in the reality of the observed state. It is the statement, "Right now this is what is important to work on."

It bears the expectation that without a decision following your observation the distance between the desired course and the current course will widen without a correction. Focus acts as your set North Star, at least for the moment, by which you can evaluate decisions.

FINDING YOUR FOCUS

Now that there is a general idea of what needs to be looked at more closely, you can begin to narrow down the specific outcome that is needed. This could be a goal for the future. It could be a solution to a problem. More than likely, it will be something that you are trying to accomplish or align to. The observe process will uncover multiple areas of possibility, and for now, deciding on just one is important. Observe could even lead you to an obvious conclusion that makes sense to focus on. You can always run through the framework another time and another time again, if needed, in order to locate the focus. Often, when you aren't certain of the focus, it's most helpful to take the best contender, that one puzzle piece, and walk it through the rest of the framework to solidify it. This is more feasible and ultimately more helpful than adding to the confusion by trying to focus on multiple puzzle pieces at once.

70

Focus is about deciding. For the small decisions it's about getting to an answer sooner rather than later. For larger decisions it is about narrowing down and chewing on the "North Star" of your life. Focus is sifting through the many pieces left from observing and panning out the gems. It's redefining and challenging yourself to reduce the many millions of possibilities to one direction that you can go … for now. It's giving yourself a decisive point to bring your future actions into some sort of order and sense.

Focus is necessary to bridge observe and act because with no focus, the action will lead to chaos and miss the specific outcome that you hope for. To further illustrate the focus step, think about brainstorming. After spending time getting all the ideas out of your head, there still is a lot of uncertainty and options to choose from. Even though you have eliminated some confusion, there is still a giant ball of information. If you tried to pursue all the items you came up with in your brainstorm at once, it would lead to a shallow engagement with each one and make little or no real movement. It would be another way to chase your tail and remain stagnant. Without a focus your efforts are spread thin and the effective outcome of the brainstorm is diluted and unsuccessful.

In reality if you have a good grasp on where you are and where you want to get to, then your time spent observing will be minimal and you can jump to focus and act.

Why is this focus step so important? As discussed previously, by eliminating extraneous factors and focusing on a single aspect, you set yourself up to most accurately land on the one single problem and one single possible solution. Just having less to decide on alleviates many issues that can cause you to procrastinate. It also helps you to quickly identify opportunities that align with your direction. Lastly it helps you to be decisive and stop the tendency to second-guess yourself or not commit to a choice.

Think about how much simpler decisions become when they are limited. In some ways we love to have choices; however, we often don't make great decisions with so many choices. Having less to chew on creates a better result from a decision because more attention is given to a few ideas and what really matters versus being spread out to too many. Even with many decisions, simply choosing between two at a time is more helpful than trying to keep our eyes on more than that.

Let me repeat: you are the only person who can determine what is right for you. There are all sorts of anxieties and concerns that come with getting ready to move in uncertain directions. In the end they won't matter. Sure, you can take note of them, but if you want to head in your truest direction, then you will have to move through them. I am confident you can and will. Focus is setting your course to follow, come hell or high water.

QUESTIONS TO HELP YOU FOCUS

- *What is important to me and what is irrelevant?*
- *Where do I currently want to get to?*
- *What am I able to control?*
- *What has worked previously for me?*
- *What is the outcome I am looking for? Will the outcome actually help me?*
- *How can this outcome be summarized clearly?*
- *Does the summary sound right? If not, what is off or missing? How will this resolve the summary statement?*
- *What other ways could this be solved?*
- *What is worth it to me to commit to?*

- *What else is needed?*
- *How will this focus align with what is meaningful to me?*

ANDREW + FOCUS

Remember in the previous chapter that Andrew and I began talking about why he got into planning? To quickly review we talked about how it was important for him to provide for his family. He shared an amazing story about working as a life insurance agent before becoming a financial planner. He had some clients that were just starting out in their life together. Unfortunately, the husband passed away unexpectedly. When the widow had no idea what to do with the insurance check, it was at that moment Andrew picked up on his why. He wanted to help people manage their money well to give them a sense of security. He spent the next five years building a business to do so. But he'd never taken the time to reflect and recognize this important truth and had never connected his way of running his business with this truth.

So as we reflected and observed, all of the observations during our meetings started working together. The observations had a few behind-the-scenes truths that were in common. There was a tension from Andrew's engagement with people. He always seemed to recognize and focus in on making sure people had a plan for their finances. He saw gaps as people discussed their intentions with their retirement. The widow, his family, and his clients all had areas where they were vulnerable, and Andrew saw it, every time. This led to him focusing in on and recognizing there was a common theme in what he regularly saw in others and what he wanted to help solve. It was providing security. As he began seeing that tension and knowing what it was, he was able to leverage it to help. In this way Andrew started to define and focus his priority in work and life.

The work behind Andrew finding his focus entailed him looking and staring long enough to notice what was meaningful and consistent in his life. If he'd never paused to observe the normal and seemingly insignificant points, the realization and the focus may have never come. As he did his observing, he became familiar enough with his current way of operating and noticed what stood out in small ways but in many places. Security didn't come as a shocker when it finally showed up as what he needed to focus on to grow his business. The shocker was that he had not yet, up to this point, actively realized it.

OTHER EXAMPLES OF FOCUS

Here is an example of another way that focus can come about. My family and I decided to head out to a local restaurant to grab dessert together. We'd skip dinner and go right to dessert. The intent was to do something a little out of the ordinary that would give us time to catch up and enjoy time together. So we headed out to a chain restaurant. We got seated pretty quickly, but the server didn't come around for about 20 minutes. Once we ordered the desserts, it took another 30 minutes. I was already frustrated and starting to lose patience. When the desserts finally arrived, the chocolate chip brownie was burnt so badly we couldn't cut it. The cheesecake was partly frozen, and one dessert didn't even get served. The entire meal experience was a disaster.

Rather than reacting to the disappointing experience, I engaged Compass Form and observed what was going on. From there, I calibrated back to the focus of the evening. The focus: we wanted to spend time together, and that was exactly what we were doing. The kids got to color, and we played chopsticks, a game the kids quickly showed us how to play. Sure, the meal was a disaster, but in that moment because the experience aligned with the focus, it had value greater than the meal. That focus allowed us to be empathetic to the situation and walk out of that experience without carrying the baggage of what could have been an extremely miserable attitude.

What this experience illustrates: not every situation coming from Compass Form will be pleasant, but being able to quickly identify your focus will allow you to find where to go next and see a greater value beyond the present circumstance.

Another example—last year I began working with the CEO of a large insurance trust. In one of our first meetings, we were observing and discussing some of the outcomes that the CEO wanted to work on. Being the leader for their organization came with many challenges and required this person to put in a lot of time to build relationships with strategic partners, the board of trustees, and employees at the company. There were many responsibilities to manage and delegate as well.

At first it sounded like this person was looking to find balance. But as we talked through what balance meant and what balance would look like, it dawned on me that balance was impossible. There would always be too many directions to be pulled or pushed into. There would always be urgent matters to give attention to. Sacrificing their health and sanity for the next opportunity would always be in tension as long as this person held that position. That burden was draining and exhausting and affecting their physical and mental capacities.

And in that observation, the focus became obvious. Balance was unattainable, but self-management was something that they could build. The real villain was that it was difficult to choose from the many opportunities, so this CEO would sacrifice their own personal life to try and create some semblance of balance. As they began to shift focus from trying to create balance to simply managing their time and energy, solutions became more apparent to them. It was similar to the airline public service announcement, "Put your mask on before helping others." When the focus shifted from trying to find balance into focusing on managing themselves better, it became clear for them how to create a better situation.

Once you have set the intention of focus, it's time to move on to the last part of Compass Form—act. Most often people are spending time thinking about their ideas and dreaming up scenarios or the "what." However, the "how to get it done" gets less time. People turn to processes and plans that have worked for others but that don't necessarily line up with them. They try and fit their idea into someone else's framework. It's like hoping your key will fit the lock to someone else's home that you saw in a magazine. In the next chapter's discussion of act, the previous steps of observe and focus ensure that when you act, you are always using your own key to unlock your own home.

SCENIC OVERLOOK

- Focus flows from the observation.
- Focus highlights and connects the common value that's at play in most of your observations.
- Focus gives you the clarity needed to fight for what is meaningful in your life.
- Focus can only come from you.
- Focus involves saying no to many things, and that is completely fine.

PERSONAL DECLINATION

- In what ways would focus be a challenge for you?
- How would finding a focus be helpful?

- What are some situations in your life where you lost focus, either by fear or distraction?
- Where could you see focus getting you through a tough circumstance?

OUT-AND-BACK EXERCISE

Take an area that you have tension or confusion around. Take a few minutes to observe. After observing, work on focusing on one outcome you'd like to head towards. Try it out as soon as possible.

- Reflect on what happened and what you experienced.
- What was difficult about focusing in?
- What did you learn about yourself or the circumstances?
- If needed, how would you refocus based on new observation and reflection?

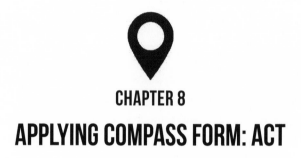

CHAPTER 8
APPLYING COMPASS FORM: ACT

"Intuition is the map to buried treasure. It is not infallible, but neither is our reason. And it can point us in the right direction. We need to pay attention to this inner voice."

—*Platform: Get Noticed in a Busy World*
by Michael Hyatt

This chapter is going to talk about the way to go about taking your observations and focus and doing something to get you closer to your greater destination. As mentioned, Compass Form is meant to be permeable. So act is less about finding the perfect plan and more about moving ahead, often by trial and error. With act, you find the next best step. If your focus turns out to be a bigger dream, then there is probably going to be a larger journey to get to your results, therefore, many steps to take. And that's fine, but act is about the next single step—not about all the next steps.

Quite often, at some point in this journey you won't know exactly where to go next. You'll see how simply taking a step (i.e., act) in the general direction of your focus produces the desired outcome, even if you don't have the best laid out picture. Again, act is not about perfection, and it's not about building the whole road to your destination. It's about the next step.

ACT OVERVIEW

Act is the final step of the framework. Without action, observe and focus become nothing more than time spent thinking. To think about the captaining a ship comparison, act is the correction we make in our steering to point us in the direction that we want. It doesn't get us there, but allows us to head in the right direction. In time as we keep the consistency of stepping (i.e., acting) in the same direction, we will draw closer to the ambition. This step allows us to slow down and see the parts of a choice and disciplines us to stay moving even when we can't totally see the right outcome. The Compass Form framework is not meant to put us at an end goal; it is meant to help us move at the pace that we were built to move in toward that end goal. To not rush through life, but not get stuck either. It is a way for us to get found when we are lost.

Often when we think about this last step, because of the work from the two previous steps, we want an action step that is foolproof. Again, that's not a helpful way to look at it. This step isn't an answer; instead, see it as providing feedback or as a point we can look at to map our progress to the destination. We can track the act step and reflect on its alignment to the steps that get us to the end goal. But we can't predict the future, so we are left in limbo to see what taking this step produces (that's the feedback part of it). There is no way around the journey, and there is nothing wrong if "success" doesn't happen immediately. But recall that if the journey isn't worth the cost, then you may have missed the right focus.

ACT IN ACTION

When we take a step of action, it isn't often we will be ready to cross the finish line or leap a canyon. More than likely we will look to make a small change. Maybe just a degree from our current direction. But think of how significant even one degree can change a course. It is similar to saving $1 dollar a day to produce $365 in a year. Without each dollar invested there would not be the same return. Hooray, if we can invest $10 or $100 per day someday, but this is about consistently acting for the same focus until we get to where we want to get to.

When you are looking to transition from focus to action, keep in mind the action should be easily attainable. It is difficult to totally release ourselves from a long-held habit, so a quick, small success will help us keep moving in the right direction. Let me note that if you never change or take any kind of action, even the smallest of actions, then you should expect the same results you previously experienced. Along the same lines, taking too big of a jump will feel very laborious and make you think you chose wrongly if you don't succeed. That's why act is about small, quick steps.

I've even noticed that as we take these steps, our original intent typically evolves into something beyond what we could fathom before starting. We are always gaining and learning, even when it's subconscious. There are new ideas and possibilities that will show up down the road as we make progress through many cycles of observe, focus, and act. For this reason, leaving space to upgrade the original idea is necessary. This is one reason it is important to be flexible with the journey. It's not an already laid-out, defined race. It's a shifting sea that you are navigating.

Another point to keep in mind is that we aren't going to know if the step is right until we take it and try it on, as much as we hope that each step is the right one. Sometimes a step can reveal other steps that need to be taken. When this happens, it may feel like two steps back, but we still learn valuable information that will inform our next cycle of observe, focus, and act.

The idea of the step is to get us moving in the right direction, long enough to find a next and better step. But all steps are steps and meant to be left behind. In this way Compass Form allows us to build flexibility and the skill to adapt once we learn something new. We become more in tune with our changing world. We align and can adjust as necessary to keep in step with the journey of the focus.

QUESTIONS TO HELP YOU ACT

- *What small action can I try to prove the observation and focus?*
- *How could this act move me closer to the focus?*
- *What will I need to change or set in place to ensure the completion of the task?*
- *How is this dependent on anyone else?*
- *What makes this act reasonable?*
- *Is this a one-time task or a habit that needs to be replaced or replace something?*
- *How can I make this more simple?*
- *What do I need to focus on to ensure success?*
- *How can I make this more achievable?*
- *What is the plan after taking this step? If none, that is fine.*

ANDREW + ACT

The way Andrew saw the world was to provide security. This, then, would be the focus for his action to change his business. For Andrew, identifying this focus uncovered what attracted clients to him. His act would be to fight to help them find security in life.

He enjoyed that work. It was his calling. Identifying our calling is the most important truth we can find for ourselves.

In the background of his week-to-week engagement with the framework of observing, focusing, and acting, Andrew identified a larger pattern cycling. And the Compass Form that helped Andrew access his week-to-week smaller action steps also uncovered a bigger life secret for him. Andrew's clients were drawn to his ability to help them grow in their financial security, and he only needed to navigate the best way to accomplish that. This truth had escaped him previously, so he'd spent his client meetings trying to figure out what to help with and how to help. Now he only had to find the way and not the what. It's like carrying two 50-pound sacks of concrete and being able to set one down. It was easy. What this looked like for Andrew: during client meetings he was freed up to listen to the client. He could see the end outcome and was free to figure out how to help his clients find it.

This one truth changed Andrew's life. It gave him a way to recognize how he shows up best in life. Not what circumstances will make him happy. But what work he will carry to every aspect of his life that will produce endless joy and satisfaction. By knowing what he was looking for, it simplified how he would approach many different situations. It eliminated some of the redundant questions and the cycle of worry Andrew had put himself through. It's a North Star that he can now always look towards when he is lost. He can now captain his ship rather than run an endless race that took him in circles and got him nowhere but frustrated.

So now Andrew uses Compass Form in his business. He observes why clients are there, focuses on what specifically they want to accomplish, and then provides the steps of action they will use to find security with their finances. Because he has a framework to follow, he is now able to give all his attention to the person directly in front of him.

Less than a year after we finished our work together, Andrew sent me an email informing me that his income from the previous year had grown by 40% as a result of our work together. As a result of Compass Form. You see, when you aren't anxious and distracted, you are free to pick up on things you might have missed. Being present for his clients not only increased his success with the clients he had, it also increased the referrals from those clients and continued to grow his business. Way to go, Andrew!

The beauty of the framework is that it isn't meant for you to keep looking at. It is meant to help you get your bearings so that you can be present to what is going on in your life. It is simple to remember, so you don't have to spend time learning how to use it. You can quickly set a course that means something to you in real time and put it away until you get turned around.

Compass Form is meant to simplify the big challenges and the smallest tasks. It helps you find where you are, where you want to go, and what you can do to take a step closer to your purpose. Life is not predictable, so having a framework provides you a go-to way to make sense of the variety so that you can take an action to move closer to your ultimate destination.

SCENIC OVERLOOK

- Act is any step in the direction of focus. It is not the result.
- Act is a trial-and-error approach to making your intentions a reality.
- Act is better with simple and feasible steps, not complicated, grandiose ones.

- Act is an investment in closing the gap between where you are and where you are heading.

PERSONAL DECLINATION

- How would focusing on a single act change how you engage with goals or problems?
- What are some of the areas that act might be a challenge to stick to?
- What would consistent acts lead to you achieving in a given area?
- What might help you to stay on course and keep with the same action?

OUT-AND-BACK EXERCISE

Think of an activity or goal that you want that has some significance for you.

- What is one act that would be useful to get a small step closer to the results of that goal?

Take the one act and make sure that each day you give five minutes of time dedicated to doing it. This could be sticking to a new habit, it could be saving money for a trip, or it could be not complaining about your job. There are so many options here!

- What did you experience this week?
- What was the end-of-the-week result of the tiny investments you made?

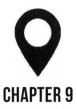

CHAPTER 9

COMPASS FORM: OBSERVE, FOCUS, ACT

"You will find peace in knowing that you will never resolve the tension—it will always be there, and there is nothing inherently wrong with it."

— Halftime: Changing Your Game Plan from Success to Significance
by Bob P. Buford

Just like my recommendation to start small with your act steps, incorporating Compass Form in your approach to life can happen in tiny bites or all at once. By isolating each phase, it will be easier to understand the whole. This chapter focuses on putting together the three phases of Compass Form and further digging into how to apply the framework to your day-to-day living.

PUTTING IT ALL TOGETHER

Think about this—the framework isn't about providing answers. Part of the benefits from this new framework is becoming content with not knowing. Typically we live in the manner of sight then faith, meaning we first want to see something and then (maybe) we'll believe it. We want proof, evidence. However, this framework requires the opposite. It requires moving without knowing and maybe for an extended period of time. Especially when we first begin, there is a lot to uncover.

At times it will feel as if you are uncovering more and more and being set back from moving ahead. This isn't so. You are uncovering all the pieces in the puzzle, which, of course, can be overwhelming. But nonetheless, whether you agree or disagree with what you see, there is no real way to get around it. If you want to bake cookies, you have to get in the kitchen and bake. You have to clean dishes, you have to buy an oven. But most often we can only see the warm cookies hitting the inside of our bellies. What this means then is that when we see more of the whole journey to arrive somewhere, it can cause us to believe something is wrong because we'd only considered the ultimate destination. However, just because we simply can't anticipate everything that we'll encounter on a journey beforehand, that doesn't mean we shouldn't try or keep going even when it gets tough. It means there is a learning curve that is unknown and whatever is worth our time better be worth the cost.

Once you take a step, and even when you don't, everything will change in at least a small way. This is a major reason that this framework is so successful. It accounts for change and anticipates that you will quickly want to gauge how to adjust once you've taken a step or two. Rather than running through an entire program or process, the framework will keep in step with your intention because you will be repeating the Compass Form cycle as needed. In a second run-through of the cycle, your observation may be to check in to see if you are on course after you've taken a tiny act step. Repeating the framework allows you to see how your steps are making an impact, and you can choose to adjust accordingly. It's like looking down at the speedometer to make sure you are going the speed that is appropriate for the road. I should add that it's likely that in time you'll get a feel for the road and your speed, and repeating the framework may not need to be as frequent.

In order to replace old habits with new ones, there will be a cost and a loss. A loss of comfort, familiarity, and a sense of knowing. But as we considered in the chapters before, losing isn't all that bad. Especially when it becomes redemption. Most often we quit before we realize the return on our investment. This framework is meant to keep us moving and investing. When we lose hope, it allows us to remember what we intended, count the cost, and move towards the direction we set out to find at the beginning. You'll always have two choices: turn back or keep going.

COMPASS FORM

Observe: the taking of an inventory of where you are right now and what is realistically possible

Focus: the single idea that aligns your observation to your desired intention

Act: the "how to" of your focus that gets you moving in the right direction

OBSERVE

What is going on right now?

What else?

What is my responsibility
and what is the responsibility
of others?

How would I want others to
approach a similar situation?

What seems to be causing the
problem or issue?

What do my feelings tell me
about the circumstance?

What other perspectives could I
look at this circumstance with?

What is missing from the
picture of my circumstances?

Is this worth the time and
energy, or should I move on?

I'll brainstorm any and all info
that comes to mind regarding
what I have been thinking
about, relevant or not.

What doesn't make sense?

What clear themes or patterns
can I see? Can the brainstorm
be organized?

I'll take a deep breath and
take one last shot at adding
something else.

FOCUS

What is important, and what is irrelevant?

Where do I currently want to get to?

What am I able to control?

What has worked previously?

What is the outcome I am looking for? Will the outcome actually help?

How can this be summarized clearly?

Does the summary sound right? If not, what is off or missing?

What other ways could this be solved?

What is worth committing to?

How will this resolve the summary statement?

What else is needed?

ACT	What small action can I try to prove the observation and focus? How could this act move me closer to the focus? What will I need to change or set in place to ensure the completion of the task? What makes this act reasonable? Is this a one-time task or a habit that needs to be replaced or replace something? How can I make this more simple? What do I need to focus on to ensure success? What is the plan after taking this step? If none, that is fine.

These pieces—observe, focus, and act—aren't made to work alone. There is a reason for each portion that builds from each previous part. Were you to use a phase on its own, it would cause a breakdown of the framework. To skip observe would be to leave out useful information that gives you a better picture of what is true. To never find focus would create confusion and uncertainty and never-ending decision-making. And to fail to act would leave you exactly where you started and no further. This next section will add some additional clarification of each phase to help identify the start and finish.

Observe—the intention is to account for where you are in life right now. It is separating how you might feel and think about your circumstances from the true nature of the circumstance.

The input is this—when you find yourself circling in thought, take time to look at the details that are coming to mind; they are there for a reason. Typically this is around stress or challenge. You can write it down or just keep track in your head. Once you have unloaded what is on your mind, you can begin sorting and organizing what seems more important and applicable to the challenge.

Example: Say, you want to start getting fit by going to a gym, but you haven't done anything about it. It's just an intention. You could engage Compass Form to figure out the best initial small step to take. In observing you might uncover the tension as involving any or several of the following: finding the time to go, wanting to go, finding a place to work out, not knowing anyone, fatigue mentally, fatigue physically, knowing that you should work out but not liking it, not knowing how to work out, not knowing how to prepare, not knowing what you need to do after a workout like where to change clothes, not liking to change in public places, having to meet strangers, not knowing how to check in.

The output is this—a few observations from your list that seem more important than others

Example: needing to choose a place to go and work out, needing to fit it into a schedule, and needing to commit

Focus—the intention is to figure out where you want to get to. This step is around narrowing down your observations to settle on a direction that makes sense right now. People are better at solving one problem at a time, so what makes the most sense to work towards right now?

The input is this—take the observations from the previous step and begin looking at what is important about the observation. Look for patterns or insights as to why these observations matter to you. Focus comes as you allow what is significant to come out of the observation.

Example: if you want to be more healthy by working out, then you have to work out. So how will you do this?

The output is this—settling on a direction or intention that makes sense in finding a solution to the problem/insight

Example: for now, where will you start to learn how to transition from someone who is not working out to someone who is working out? While there are many right choices here, the point is not to find the single right one. The point is to find one that makes sense and try it out.

Act—the intention is to find a simple action to move you closer to the result you want. This step is about taking an idea and making a real change to affect your circumstances.

The input is this—find an easy step that touches on a few of the observations and is in line with the focus.

Examples:
Commit to working out for a year. *Honestly, this act step is too big and too generic.*

Download seven workout plans and try them out. *This act step is too complicated and a huge expenditure on resources and energy.*

Put workout clothes by the door. *This act step is too small and shortsighted.*

Call a gym close by and ask for a walk-through. *This one might be just right.*

Find a friend who is currently doing consistent workouts and ask to join up. *This might also be just right.*

The output is this—take a step to get you moving to where you want to go. You may not know if this step is right or wrong until you take it, but you will have learned more about what mattered to you and have a better idea in the future of what you are intending to accomplish.

Hopefully what you can see in the given example is that by applying Compass Form to your situation you quickly move from chaos and confusion to making a sensible decision that will change something in your life. It helps you to identify from all the clutter what is currently important and will lead you to getting closer to what matters, even when you're not certain on exactly what that is yet. It breaks down any complexity into a simple and tangible action. When you combine consistent steps, your intention stays true and the end aligns with what you wanted to see happen.

REPEAT

It is worth noting that there is a final part to the framework that we mentioned when we talked about doing many cycles of the framework. We can call this repeat. Since there are multiple steps between where you are starting and where you want to get to, there will be times to return back to Compass Form to cycle through it again in order to confirm you are still on track, to find the next step to act on, or to adjust the course as needed. This isn't a set-it-and-forget-it plan of action. Every once in a while, or in some instances—quite often—it makes sense to look at the compass and get your bearings, so you don't end up too far down the highway before realizing you missed your exit.

As I've worked with clients to both hone the framework and help them achieve goals, I'll share a few stories—first one about James, then one about George, and a final one about me—to further bring home how the framework empowers people. In reading these notice the changes in perspective and how Compass Form relates to your story.

JAMES + COMPASS FORM

James was always full of life and looking for the next opportunity to have a good time and to have a good time with as many people as possible. He had a huge smile and a warm and welcoming personality. It was a shock to sit down and chat with a guy that looked like he was winning at life and hear that it wasn't all that others could see from the outside. You never really know what goes on in other people's lives until you ask.

James came to me with a major problem. He had been working in the credit union industry for many years and left that platform to join an emerging company. It wasn't going well. He was in the sales side of using his past relationships to propose a new product for the credit unions to offer to their members. As we began meeting, he shared what was currently going on with his work.

In doing our observation step we took account of the pain points that kept showing up. He was so busy trying to achieve that he'd become disconnected from his own life. He wasn't seeing the results he expected or the ones he needed. It was getting to the point where if James didn't change, he might lose the dream of building the business. The problem was that he was busy as hell meeting with clients but not getting the sale.

James hadn't hit bonus really since joining the team a few years before and the lack of income was affecting his work, his marriage, and himself. Just before we started to work together, he was pulled into a conversation with his boss and was for the most part put on probation and was edging too close to losing his job.

The problems we uncovered by taking a look at what was happening were ones he had been trying to work on for years. His tendency was to over-promise and get stuck trying to fulfill the commitments that resulted from over-promising. This was a repetitive habit that went unseen and was the major contributor to the lack of results he was seeing. He was amazing at managing and softening the mistakes that contributed to his lack of results. He is and was a phenomenal showman, effortlessly giving off the perception that everything was okay. But under that cover, life wasn't okay, and James was quickly finding that there was no air left to breathe.

So we began to work together to get to the bottom of where he was: observe. The first and most important part of his process was to locate the problem: observe and focus. On the surface the lack of income, the stress that created, and the disappointment were very clear. As he shared, we could dig a little more to make sure that we even touched on parts that seemed irrelevant.

James was working hours beyond a healthy level to try and make up for the lack of results. This created a limited amount of time for the rest of life, which caused him to try harder and shortened his patience. He was panicking and losing his head at coworkers, his family, and mostly at himself. It was a cycle that had been building for years and became the perfect storm that had to be navigated. His pain was affecting his life in almost every capacity.

So as we **observed** his routines and habits, he began to see the truth of the matter. When a person says things aloud, something special happens. Typically we don't say what isn't true, and there was hesitation in James's voice when he described the scenarios. He was able to quickly begin recognizing and **focusing** on the problem: he was trying way too hard even though, in fact, he was not aware of what needed to be done. He believed if he just worked a little harder, that would eventually fix the problem. He was managing the problem but not addressing it. He knew he was running out of time and couldn't keep up anymore.

James also found that he was really talking about the symptoms of the problem. The real problem was underneath what he was seeing and frustrated with. We had to find what was creating the symptoms. As we **observed** a little more, some new information began to show up: when he didn't get a sale, he believed it was because he'd done something incorrectly and must try harder and prepare more for the next one. This added to more time and pressure with having to invest into work. This was leading to over-promising clients with deadlines and follow-up. It led to additional work that he didn't have time for, which, in turn, created more stress, worry, and a short temper.

But he didn't have time to organize or take a step back and look at other ways. The more things didn't work, the more he would put his head down to charge ahead. His natural skills and gifts were being eaten away by his fear of this dream not working out.

The end observation turned into the beginning of the **focus**. Here is what we uncovered. When James looked at what the future might hold, he got nervous when looking at the obstacles that were keeping him from getting to the end goal. He lost sight of what he was currently capable of and tried to will the future to work out. Instead of focusing on what he could do right now, he would be anxious about life not working out the way he hoped. He was spending so much time not present to what he could actually affect.

He would start a project and not really finish it. So the proposals couldn't be sent out, and he would miss the self-imposed deadlines. Those items kept adding up and creating even more pressure that kept him from being as successful as he could be.

Through our conversations James uncovered that his fear of the future not working out was driving him to panic and lose sight of obvious places to improve. He had to find another way because this way had been failing for a while. We discussed **focusing** on what he could control at work in the present. He saw that he had a list of items that needed to get done. We also worked on how to work through the backlog of items that were piling up and also how to keep from creating more unfinished items.

Previously when James got anxious, he would look to add more value, even though the clients didn't ask for or need this additional value. Next he wouldn't follow up or through with clients because he'd over-promised. So he started with a new focus: to stay aware of what needed to get done. It was a general focus, but it was effective enough to allow him to align his choices with his focus.

Rather than committing to getting a quote out the next day, James would only promise to follow up with a quote. Not having to carry the added pressure of timing allowed him to complete action items and not lose track when something that he forgot came to mind.

He found that as he reduced the unnecessary promises, he began to reduce some of the burden he was carrying, and this freed up his mind for more insights.

So he started to take one thing at a time. We built a schedule to work on what needed to get done today and then with what time was left over, James would work on the backlog. He could begin to see how a plan would help free him from the burden in his mind of what he needed to do, what would happen if he didn't, and what he would need to do if the worst happened.

As James kept with the plan, we started seeing immediate results. James was able to send proposals out on time; the backlog, though not completely gone, was shrinking. In just our first month working together, James hit a bonus for the first time. His boss even pulled him aside to congratulate him on his reversal of attitude and great results. The coworkers he managed benefitted from his better responses too.

James saw that simple and consistent effort in a **focused** direction led him to the success he had wanted all along. He observed that when life became a little chaotic, he would become overwhelmed. Rather than slowing down to get a good look at what was contributing to the chaos, he would add more tasks to complete.

From there James only had to start with remembering one thing. When he got overwhelmed, he would take a look at what was going on and then record items on a list. He would get items out of his head, which allowed him to focus on what he needed to get done now. And then he was able to get the task he was currently working on completed.

Another change with James' family is worth noting. Soon after James saw the dramatic changes happening in his life, he also began to see the world differently. The release of tension from work was starting to play out in other areas of his life.

While preparing to go to a concert with his wife, James had a really brilliant insight. From what I understand, getting ready to go out was not always smooth. And on this evening there were some delays on getting out the door, and the typical tension was starting to build. But James **observed** it coming and found a new way. Rather than venting about his frustration, he **focused** enough to ask a question. He asked his wife why it was so important to look the part before going out. Her answer was not what he expected. She mentioned it was for him, and that she didn't believe that he would want to be with her if she didn't.

Since that was obviously not the case, it was easy for James to **act**. He responded that he didn't want that from her. He loved her the way she was. But because they had made some assumptions, that truth had never come out. So they would work hard at what they thought the other found important rather than asking.

That night there was a big shift in their relationship. Because James could now see that he wasn't participating with the relationship and he was making assumptions there as well. The only real shift—the **act**—that was needed was for him to take the time to be present. He learned that the truth would show up when he slowed down to look for it. Life didn't have to be "fixed" or made "right" in order to be present.

James was slowing down enough to observe situations for simple details. And those details were how he got big results. He made note of what he saw and focused on a pattern that he could change. And then he took a small step to make that change.

This was James's big lesson that showed up. His results were incredible, and they appeared within our first month of working together. Typically clients agree to work together with me for three months, and we hope by the end of those three months some positives begin to emerge, but James was far ahead of this timeline. By the end of that year he was hitting the bonus at work and enjoying his home life too. Again, I invite you to contact me to explore our working together, so I can help you to orient yourself to what matters most to you as well: jacob@themountainpassway.com and https://themountainpassway.com.

GEORGE + COMPASS FORM

When I first met George, he was still picking up the pieces from a relationship that ended. The rest of his life was not as problematic. He was a guy who has seen the results of working hard and became a leader in his industry. But after the relationship ended, George became lost. This broken relationship began to compound with other personal matters that brought about a depressive state that George would go in and out of. All the added stress eventually became too much to handle on his own. And so we agreed to start working together.

It took a while for us to work through the many layers of complexity. There was a lot of listening to **observe** and then **focus** to determine what the issue was and how to work out of it. We used a phenomenal tool called the Enneagram, which helps you see how you tend to engage and how you might see the world reveal itself to you. Here is a snippet from the analysis of George's Enneagram. George was best characterized as the following: "Considerate Helper— someone who wants to meet others' needs in a helpful, supportive way. Warm, giving, and people-oriented, they seek affirmation from their relationships and may be sensitive and angry if they feel unappreciated. They may over-involve themselves in others' lives and risk being manipulative. Their development challenge is to give unconditionally and to nurture themselves as well as others."

Because of George's way of engaging in his personal relationships, more specifically the one that ended so painfully, he was financially taken advantage of because of his generosity. This turned the relationship sour. He would give, and she would take. His personality was to be supportive, and this vulnerability, when left unattended, opened an easy way to be misused.

Now there are two sides to the coin. George enjoyed helping others, but he also found a bit of his identity in it. The way it would work is that as he would give—and here's the other side of the coin—to him it was like he was investing in a bank account that he could withdraw from. This had been his approach for a long while. It was both a blessing and a curse for him.

So he would give to others, both for his own benefit as well as theirs. The problem became that when he didn't get recognized for the effort, he'd get angry at the person he gave to. Eventually he would forgive the person in his own mind, but the cycle would continue. He would give and give, and there would not be a reciprocation or at least at the value he had hoped for. At some point this became too much, and while this one particular significant relationship ended, how he engaged the world didn't. He would still give to get.

In George's case we used the Enneagram tool to help **observe** what he was immediately experiencing and also expose the long-standing pattern. For George the **observation** led to a revelation, which became his **focus** that he would take small steps to **act** on: he wasn't taking care of his own needs because he concentrated on giving attention to others. He was drowning at the expense of trying to be supportive to others.

If you have been paying attention throughout the book, you can already predict the story from here. I could end it here, and you could figure out what happened next. It shows how when you **observe** thoroughly, it can become easy to locate the core problem. With that **focus**, the solution, i.e., how to **act**, becomes apparent. You know exactly what to **focus** on and how to **act**. That doesn't mean it will be an easy road, but it eliminates the confusion and opens the truth up so that you deal accurately.

With this **focus** George was able to start recognizing areas in his life where this particular perspective was noticeable. He began to invest in himself—so this is where he would **act**—where he had previously neglected. He began focusing on finding some intentions to build on to better himself, like eating healthier and paying off some debt. These **actions** came from identifying the accurate **focus**, which was the need to care for himself. He is continuing to build a life that means a lot to him without the tension to sacrifice his own requirements for the sake of others.

ME AGAIN + COMPASS FORM

After running for a few years, I started getting into racing. I enjoyed running and liked the steady improvements that came from working hard and showing up regularly. I found a great group to help make the time on my feet a little easier. I was running some 5ks, 10ks, and half marathons. I started at over a 30-minute 5k, and after working on different forms and ways to train, eventually I was running a 5k under 21 minutes.

Running is a good teacher, and you can't cheat running. You have to put the time in to see results. In 2018, I was becoming a little bored with road races and started looking into trail running and mountain running. There is a mountain in New Hampshire that is pretty special in my life: Mt. Washington at 6,288 feet and home to the world's worst weather. For New England that is one of the highest peaks, and as a kid I remember driving up the auto-road and spending time at the top checking out the observatory and historic buildings. Since then I've probably hiked up it at least ten times. And when I found a race that went up the 7.6 miles of the auto-road to the top, I naively signed up for the lottery to win a bib.

Without knowing whether I'd get entered into the race, I knew I had to prepare for that day, and this was the start of **observe**. So I started researching to find tips to running up hills. I was able to piece together a rough plan to get myself in shape. The race is 7.6 miles at an average of 12% grade, which is basically maxing out a treadmill to the highest incline. The final section is actually 22%. My **focus** was that if I could run for an hour and a half at 15% grade on a treadmill, then I would be close to what I needed to finish.

So I started one day a week **acting** on the intention. I remember the first time getting on the treadmill and setting that incline and trying to run. I got maybe five minutes into the run and had to stop.

I had been running for years, and I was out of breath. My first step revealed so much about this unknown journey and what it would cost me to succeed. I quickly **repeated** the framework and adjusted the **action**. I would run for as long as I could and then walk until I caught my breath. I maybe got 40 minutes into the first attempt, and maybe 10 minutes of it was actually running. This challenge was way more than I'd anticipated, but if I wanted to do the race, then I knew I would have to stay **focused** to continue. The mountain wouldn't care if I liked it or not. There is no way to get around the 4,654 feet of elevation to see the top.

Running hills is different than running flatter roads. In time I grew stronger and the minutes I could run at that grade grew. By the time the race came I was running well over an hour at that incline. I had committed to the race, and it changed my **focus** for each run. I started looking for hills to climb on easy and long runs. I would run with the group and during the run shoot off to get another hill in. In all this prep, I wasn't sure what to expect on race day. I listened to what people shared online, asked others for advice, but nothing could have prepared me to run the race without actually running it. I didn't know what I didn't know. And when race day came, I had put in the amount of time and effort that I could manage. What I didn't account for was what the race actually would be like.

After the gun set off, the entire group set out to take on the mountain. Months of many consistent **acts** and preparation finally were realized. For the first few miles I felt really good, but I could already feel my legs burning. Surely there would be a break in the climb? I had driven the road up the mountain before and never realized there was never a break from the grade. They joke that it is only one hill, and it is literally true. There is never a point in the race where the incline is under 10%.

There were a few other factors that I didn't know to account for. One was the heat. Typically in June the weather might be warm, but on this day it was even warmer than usual at around 70 degrees. So, beautiful but not ideal racing temperatures. The second factor was altitude. Running at 2,000 feet is different than running at 6,000 feet. The air thins and the oxygen mixture decreases, so breathing is more of a challenge. Lesson learned and experience gained.

By mile three I had to start walking. I was disappointed, for the goal was to run the race without walking. I never could have anticipated the experience without having it. So I walked and then tried to run. I could run for 15 seconds and then would have to walk, and the breaks between running were getting longer.

So I had to make an **observation** in the moment and find a new **focus**. It was tragic to have to let go of a goal and not run the race in the way I envisioned—but I was "captaining a ship" and had to "adjust course," according to the real-time conditions. So I resigned to walking the rest of the way. I would try a few more times to run, but as I gained elevation, I didn't have the lungs or energy needed. But in resigning, I **refocused** to find another way to finish. I noticed that I could hike faster than I could jog. I was beginning to pass people that had passed me. And my **observation** in that moment had helped me to adapt to a new possibility. It turned out to be a good decision, but I had no idea at the moment. I was able to take in the race in a different light.

As a kid I remembered days at the top where the clouds were so thick I couldn't see my fingers in front of my face. But that day was clear, and I could see the world. In between the burning muscles I could take in parts of the race I would have missed. Not a bad consolation prize. In the end I finished that climb in under two hours, and it's a memory that reflected much of this framework that I have carried with me and lessons that I can share with others now.

There was no one to tell me I did this race "right" or that I "should have" run the race. There was no past experience that kept me from finishing. There was no dream that would have pulled me up the mountain. There was the truth of the matter. I needed every step that I took before I stepped across the start line to get myself across the finish line. No one step was more important than the next. Each step brought its own challenge. But the journey I took eventually got me to where I wanted to go.

As you can see, in the cases of James, George, and me, as well as all the examples you've read so far in this book, Compass Form provides a consistent way to avoid living in a reactionary manner. It is being aware of how you want to engage people and circumstances. Observe, focus, and act allows you a way to slow down just enough to notice more in real time but not get stuck in thinking about what to do and being paralyzed with inaction. It also helps you avoid unhealthy ruts and disengagement. Remember, Compass Form is not meant to determine the best course of action with no variants. It's meant to be a process in which a good course of action can be taken, to give you awareness and hopefully result in attentiveness to the bigger picture so that you can take a step deliberately in the direction of what matters most to you.

SCENIC OVERLOOK

- Compass Form is meant to create a rapid flow from confusion to clarity.
- Compass Form allows you to identify whether you are on course, what is next, and how to adjust.

- Compass Form simplifies complexity to give you a better understanding of your journey.
- Compass Form adapts to short-term and long-term needs.
- Compass Form bridges the gap between where you are and where you want to be.

PERSONAL DECLINATION

- What are some situations in your life that might benefit from a little attention?
- How can you see using Compass Form to make sense of a confusing situation?
- What past situations have you seen break down from your inability to see the problem? How might they have changed if you'd applied Compass Form?

OUT-AND-BACK EXERCISE

Think back to a previous experience that didn't work out so well.

- Try and create the milestones of what happened.
- Identify where, when, and how you could have implemented Compass Form to create a better outcome.

It's important to not regret or judge the outcome when reflecting on a previous approach. The exercise is about seeing the difference in approach, so you can learn and grow.

- How would you approach the same circumstance using what you have gained so far?

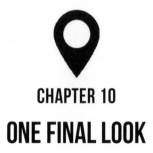

CHAPTER 10

ONE FINAL LOOK

"In pursuing one's way, the lighter one travels the better."

—*The Reformed Pastor*
by Richard Baxter

So what does success look like from the vantage point of Compass Form? Is it unicorns pooping out rainbows and pies in the sky raining down ease and success? Probably not. As I've already stated, with Compass Form success isn't about always seeing optimal results. Success is being confident that if you stay the course, you'll get to where you want to go. There's no magic wand or quick fix in life. There's always a journey. There's always a gap between where we're at and where we hope to be. We are meant to evolve and live in constant growth. In time I think we can reconcile our constant but impossible yearning to see the future, get much better at living with uncertainty, and trust that we can always make our situations better.

Success is knowing you are moving in the right direction and trusting that that's enough. How does the framework allow you to do this? It gives you a quick check-in with your current standing and where you are pointed. Once you see where you have been investing your time and resources, you can clearly see your current direction. Having an accurate direction allows you to narrow down your many options by eliminating the options that don't fit well. Think about looking at a compass. When you know where the needle should be pointed, you can eliminate three other quadrants. That's a 75% elimination just by a quick glance down.

From there everything in front of you is fair game. Since the goal isn't to figure out the exact plan and route, but just the next step, you can trust that even though you don't see the end yet, you can focus on where to land your foot next. This makes it easier to avoid holes that you might fall into when you're overly concentrated on reaching the finish. It allows you to be present to what you are responsible to right now.

Success also comes in the form of your being able to deal with uncertainty. If you aren't looking for the imaginary picture and instead looking to work with what you have and know, your confidence will grow as well as your skills to handle new situations. You become comfortable that you can handle the unknown. Uncertainty becomes an expected reality for you to handle. Choosing to make adjustments that will allow you to ultimately stay the course will produce the success you anxiously await.

If you have a question or an idea, or you'd like to explore the possibility of working with me to help you engage Compass Form in your own life, please contact me—jacob@themountainpassway.com and https://themountainpassway.com. I am available to help out.

GENEROSITY—THE ROI OF SUCCESS

So what is at the end of success and what does all this produce in our lives? Success produces generosity. When our existence isn't tied to every disruption, we can more quickly move to addressing the root problem and being effective in the handling of that. We are less sidetracked and "in need" of desperately finding solutions. When we begin to eliminate the anxious feeling of need, generosity wells. It leaves us with more to give to others. We are free to be generous even when we don't have much to give when the sense of need is reduced. We know that our time will come, and we don't have to be completely full in order to give. This is like splitting a half of a peanut butter and jelly sandwich with a friend, knowing you can grab something else later on. If you feel like you are starving, you're never giving up a bite. But when you aren't handcuffed by the sense of need, the opportunity to give freely rises up.

Success is knowing that you can use what you have, that you have the ability to grow and get what might be needed, and the patience to hold off until later. A more long-term solution. Generosity isn't based on having everything and then giving to others. Generosity is about knowing you don't have everything, don't need everything, and being able to hand out what you are capable of and that being enough.

I think deep down within we each would rather contribute and help others, but our own survival can seem insurmountable and immeasurable when we operate through the running-a-race-approach. We find ourselves only focusing on taking care of ourselves. We don't believe that others will be generous to help our needs or want to lend a hand to help us out, so we take on double duty of taking care of ourselves. Only if there is something left over, then we might give it to someone else.

Success through Compass Form places us outside of this desperation paradigm. It gives us the freedom to not allow our circumstances to control our decisions and to push ahead to the more meaningful direction we believe in. It allows us to take on the short-term cost of being uncertain and give to others despite our own sense of need. We are free to choose and initiate the life we want and no longer held captive by imagined dire futures. We can head out in a new adventure because we are not tied to the old way of being comforted or satisfied.

The gap of uncertainty between where we are and what we hope for will never close. As we realize the dreams of yesterday, they will be replaced with ideas of another more improved life. The desire to improve is a wonderful gift when held in good light. This constant tension is necessary to help us survive. All good things grow old and pass on in our life. We will have seasons that are similar. It can be hard to let go of the pieces that have shown great value in the past but that will restrict us today and tomorrow when we aren't sure of what is next. This constant need to adapt is better accomplished with Compass Form because it's a framework that allows us to exist in real time and simplify the many choices we will need to make. Rather than keeping our heads down to what is changing, we can look to make the adjustments that make sense in the moment.

With Compass Form you can maintain what matters most to you top of mind. It guides you to understand how your life has changed so that you don't wake up one day wondering how you traveled off-course and wasted your life. It's a simple, flexible, and universal framework to check in with yourself. Compass Form allows you to find your bearings when uncertainty shows up and your life shifts. It's an incredibly effective tool to put to use Before You Begin a new journey or before you take the next step on your current one.

NEXT STEPS—*FREE* COMPASS FORM EMAIL COURSE!

I welcome you to sign up to access the free email course that further guides and challenges you in engaging Compass Form in your life.

For more information and to sign up, please go here: https://themountainpassway.com/emailcourse

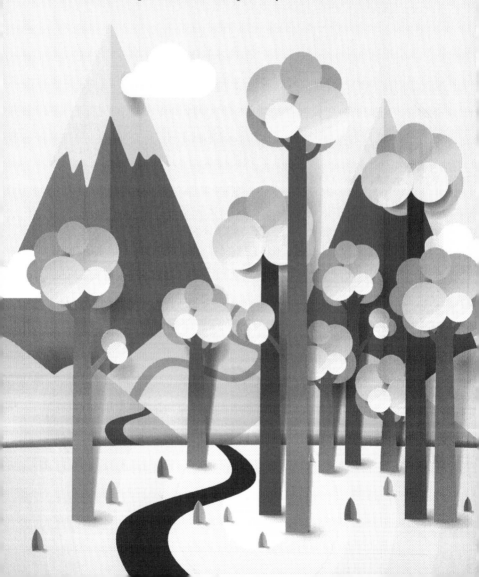

ACKNOWLEDGMENTS

Kristin Coldwell—you made this possible. Your support makes our countless hours learning together fly by. There is no person that I would rather share life with. This wouldn't have happened without you. I love you to no end.

McKenzie, Ezra, and Ezekiel—this book and message are dedicated to you. I hope it helps guide you through the obstacles and opportunities to come. It has helped me be a better dad to you. Love you all.

Art and Pam Coldwell—thank you for investing in my life and showing me a great example to follow. There is much in life that is not in our control, and I am so fortunate to be your son.

Mac Coldwell—best uncle ever and a better-than-average brother!

Mike Davis—many miles run and many ideas shared. The good thing about me getting slower is that there is more time to chat. You are a great friend, and I'll see you on Saturday.

Tyler Dunphy—a decade of work together that built the foundation of this project. Thank you, my friend, for the bottomless time with coffee.

Steve and Lori Robertson—the selfless examples that showed me how to live well. Your friendship and guidance have been immeasurable. And, yes, I am crying while writing this.

Ken Micucci—the partner in painting that slogged through the muck with me. I'd have failed without you. You are the best bud.

Steve Nevers—a good man you are, Steve Nevers. A master of the trade. Thank you for sharing your knowledge, friend.

Dan Hoffman—the true winter warrior. Thank you for the many miles run.

John McArthur—mentor and friend. Thanks for opening up your life and giving.

Don Coldwell—only a cousin, but like a brother, always.

Nancy Pile—you are a hero in this excursion. The gaps you fill and expertise you give are incredible to benefit from. Thank you for your patience and guidance.

RESOURCES FOR CONTINUED STUDY

I am a huge believer in listening to what others have taken the time to write down. These resources are meant to give you some additional places to further develop what matters to you. At some point in time each author has influenced my own development and journey.

The 5 Second Rule: Transform Your Life, Work, and Confidence with Everyday Courage
Mel Robbins

12 Rules for Life: An Antidote to Chaos
Jordan B. Peterson

All Is Grace: A Ragamuffin Memoir
Brennan Manning

Am I Making Myself Clear?: Secrets of the World's Greatest Communicators
Terry Felber

Atomic Habits: An Easy and Proven Way to Build Good Habits and Break Bad Ones
James Clear

Be Expert with Map and Compass
Bjorn Kjellstrom

Blink: The Power of Thinking Without Thinking
Malcolm Gladwell

Brimstone: The Art and Act of Holy Nonjudgment
Hugh Halter

*Building a StoryBrand: Clarify Your Message So Customers
Will Listen*
Donald Miller

*The Bullet Journal Method: Track the Past, Order the Present, Design
the Future*
Ryder Carroll

*Communication: Emotional Intelligence: The EQ Mastery
Manual—EQ, Problem Solving, Social Psychology, Social Skills*
Robert L. Kauffman

*Conversational Intelligence: How Great Leaders Build Trust and Get
Extraordinary Results*
Judith E. Glaser

Crush It!: Why NOW Is the Time to Cash In on Your Passion
Gary Vaynerchuk

*The Cry of the Soul: How Our Emotions Reveal Our Deepest
Questions About God*
Dan B. Allender

Death by Living: Life Is Meant to Be Spent
N. D. Wilson

Decisive: How to Make Better Choices in Life and Work
Chip Heath

Deep Listening: Impact Beyond Words
Oscar Trimboli

Depression: Looking Up from the Stubborn Darkness
Edward T. Welch

*Design Your Day: Be More Productive, Set Better Goals, and Live
Life On Purpose*
Claire Diaz-Ortiz

Digital Minimalism: Choosing a Focused Life in a Noisy World
Cal Newport

Drive: The Surprising Truth About What Motivates Us
Daniel H. Pink

*Emotional Intelligence for Entrepreneurs: How to Use the Secrets of
Emotional Intelligence to Achieve Better Sales, Increase EQ, Improve
Leadership, and Skyrocket the Profits of Your Business*
Joel E. Winston

*Essential Wilderness Navigation: A Real-World Guide to
Finding Your Way Safely in the Woods With or Without A Map,
Compass or GPS*
Craig Caudill

Everlasting Man
G. K. Chesterton

Finding Your Way Without Map or Compass
Harold Gatty

*Free to Focus: A Total Productivity System to Achieve More by
Doing Less*
Michael Hyatt

The Furious Longing of God
Brennan Manning

*Good Leaders Ask Great Questions: Your Foundation for Successful
Leadership*
John C. Maxwell

Halftime: Changing Your Game Plan from Success to Significance
Bob Buford

How People Change
Timothy S. Lane

How to Talk So People Will Listen
Steve Brown

*How to Write Copy That Sells: The Step-By-Step System for More
Sales, to More Customers, More Often*
Ray Edwards

How Will You Measure Your Life?
Clayton M. Christensen

If I Understood You, Would I Have This Look on My Face?: My Adventures in the Art and Science of Relating and Communicating
Alan Alda

The Inside-Out Revolution: The Only Thing You Need to Know to Change Your Life Forever
Michael Neill

The Little Book of Results: A Quick Guide to Achieving Big Goals
Jamie Smart

Living the Resurrection: The Risen Christ in Everyday Life
Eugene H. Peterson

The Lost Art of Listening, Second Edition: How Learning to Listen Can Improve Relationships
Michael P. Nichols

Man's Search for Meaning
Viktor E. Frankl

The Meaning of Marriage: Facing the Complexities of Commitment with the Wisdom of God
Timothy Keller

Mindset Makeover: Understand the Neuroscience of Mindset, Improve Self-Image, Master Routines for a Whole New Mind, and Reach your Full Human Potential
Som Bathla

The Missing Link
Sydney Banks

Narrative Coaching: The Definitive Guide to Bringing New Stories to Life
David B. Drake

Neuroscience and Critical Thinking: Understand the Hidden Pathways of Your Thought Patterns—Improve Your Memory, Make Rational Decisions, Tune Down Emotional Reactions, and Set Realistic Expectations
Albert Rutherford

A Place of Healing: Wrestling with the Mysteries of Suffering, Pain, and God's Sovereignty
Joni Eareckson Tada

The Power of Habit: Why We Do What We Do in Life and Business
Charles Duhigg

The Power of Presence: Unlock Your Potential to Influence and Engage Others
Kristi Hedges

Praying Backwards: Transform Your Prayer Life by Beginning in Jesus' Name
Bryan Chapell

Procrastinate on Purpose: 5 Permissions to Multiply Your Time
Rory Vaden

A Quest for More: Living for Something Bigger Than You
Paul David Tripp

Quiet: The Power of Introverts in a World That Can't Stop Talking
Susan Cain

The Reformed Pastor
Richard Baxter

The Relationship Handbook: A Simple Guide to Satisfying Relationships

George Pransky

Resonate: Present Visual Stories That Transform Audiences
Nancy Duarte

The Road Back to You: An Enneagram Journey to Self-Discovery
Ian Morgan Cron

Secrets of Dynamic Communications: Prepare with Focus, Deliver with Clarity, Speak with Power
Ken Davis

Seeing Through the Fog: Hope When Your World Falls Apart
Ed Dobson

Seeing with New Eyes
David Powlison

Simply Said: Communicating Better at Work and Beyond
Jay Sullivan

Speaking Truth in Love: Counsel in Community
David Powlison

Sprint: How to Solve Big Problems and Test New Ideas in Just Five Days
Jake Knapp

The Systems Thinker—Analytical Skills: Level Up Your Decision Making, Problem Solving, and Deduction Skills. Notice The Details Others Miss.
Albert Rutherford

Talk to Me: How to Ask Better Questions, Get Better Answers, and Interview Anyone Like a Pro
Dean Nelson

They Ask, You Answer: A Revolutionary Approach to Inbound Sales, Content Marketing, and Today's Digital Consumer
Marcus Sheridan

Thinker's Guide to the Art of Socratic Questioning
Richard Paul

This Is Marketing: You Can't Be Seen Until You Learn to See
Seth Godin

Tribe of Mentors: Short Life Advice from the Best in the World
Timothy Ferriss

What Got You Here Won't Get You There: How Successful People Become Even More Successful
Marshall Goldsmith

What's Wrong with the World
G. K. Chesterton

When Helping Hurts: How to Alleviate Poverty Without Hurting the Poor ... and Yourself
Brian Fikkert

Why Don't We Listen Better? Communicating and Connecting in Relationships
James C. Petersen

Wilderness Navigation: Finding Your Way Using Map, Compass, Altimeter and GPS
Bob Burns

Writing to Be Understood: What Works and Why
Anne Janzer

ABOUT THE AUTHOR

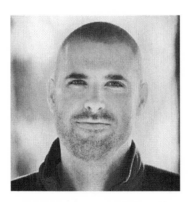

Jacob Coldwell enjoys his time helping people uncover a more meaningful life. He wrote this book and appreciates that you are reading the author bio.

For over 12 years Jacob learned many lessons from running a successful home painting service until leaving it behind (finally) to work as a certified life coach. His current profession involves guiding entrepreneurs, small business owners, and leaders to overcome obstacles and focus on what matters.

He resides in Maine with wife, Kristin, three children, and their dog, Cadence, a Jack Russell and Chihuahua mix that obviously includes another breed because she's around 25 pounds.

To learn more about Jacob Coldwell, the coaching he offers, and Compass Form, go to https://themountainpassway.com. Jacob welcomes you to contact him with questions, ideas, and also inquiries about his coaching services—jacob@themountainpassway.com.

Can You Help?

Thank You for Reading My Book!

I really appreciate all of your feedback, and
I love hearing what you have to say.

I need your input to make the next version of
this book and my future books better.

Please leave me an honest review on Amazon letting
me know what you thought of the book.

Thanks so much!

Jacob

Made in the USA
Coppell, TX
12 February 2023

12724913R00081